TAO OF INTERNAL ALCHEMY

by

Barefoot Doctor

Activating the immortal self

WAYWARD PUBLICATIONS

First published 2001 as 'Return of the Urban Warrior' by Harper Collins Publishers

This edition published by Wayward Publications Ltd © 2017 Edinburgh

www.waywardpublications.com

Cover design Spanky Pymm

British Library Cataloguing-in-Publication Data

ISBN 978-1-912062-30-0 in epub format

ISBN 978-1-912062-31-7 in mobi format

ISBN 978-1-912062-32-4 in azw3 format

ISBN 978-1-912062-33-1 in pdf format

ISBN 978-1-912062-34-8 in print

A word from the author

This is a reprinted updated version of Return of the Urban Warrior. However, owing to modern technology it is now exceedingly easy to adjust manuscript mid-flight. We therefore still welcome any feedback on references, items or chunks that, in your opinion, need updating, and we can change it accordingly – and in return the author will reward you with an acknowledgment in the revised version.

BEFORE SEEING ITS FACE (PREFACE)

Everything in the book you are about to read is based on Taoism. Though Taoism is ancient Oriental in origin, it has been generously passed down as a universally applicable system of self-development. Taoism is not a religion. It is merely a collection of methods for self-enlightenment. It will not, therefore, induce you to inadvertently or otherwise contravene the terms or tenets of any faith you currently hold dear to, either by birth or adoption. In line with the non-traditional, non-Sinophilic attitude of the author, phonetically spelled Chinese terminology has been kept to a bare minimum to avoid unnecessary confusion and instead substituted with the author's own zany, yet as-literal-as-possible translations. It is hoped this will not offend purists. But if it does, they know what they can go and do.

There are many ways to look at a book – upside down, the right way up, from a distance or up close. You can see it as a pile of sixty-odd-thousand words stuffed into a small cubic mass of solid paper matter. You can see it as the pointless destruction of yet another forest. You can see it as a worthy object to display on your shelf to close the gap between other books. You can see it as a method of escape from the perceived drudgery of daily life. You can see it as a new pile of data for your mind to absorb and store for further use. Or you can see it as a mind-altering substance – equal in potency to any strong drug of your choice. A drug that through its ingestion actually reconstitutes your reality at a radical level.

Though from my point of view as author in this particular charade (of you playing reader, me playing author), this book is written with maximum entertainment factor in mind, you could probably be far more easily entertained reading fiction or watching a movie. However, what this book promises is an interactive, somatic experience, whereby you, playing the role of reader, are led along a pathway of thought as dictated by me, playing the role of author; the very following of which will actually reconstitute your reality, or at least your experience of it, quite fundamentally.

In other words, without doing anything more than reading the contained text in sequential order, you will be taken through a transformational process which could easily result in your absolute enlightenment. And all you have to do is read it.

Like taking a pill, this text can transform you both in the short term, while reading, and indefinitely – though this transformation requires nothing more from you than your undivided attention from start to end of the text. In short, the perfect high-speed spiritual fix for people on the run.

These days we have grown accustomed to sound bites of information requiring only a very short attention span. For this chunk of information (mostly consisting of a deeply guided meditational journey of sorts) to penetrate and do its work properly though, you will need to exercise a considerably longer stretch of attention. But then who said I had to make it easy?

I do however help you concentrate by the liberal use of subtle hypnotic triggers, which enable you to relax into the process, making it an altogether painless, indeed potentially a sublimely pleasurable experience.

Incidentally, I would like to point out (especially to readers in litigation-happy societies), that when attempting anything suggested in this book, you do so by your own cognizance and that neither I, the book's publishers, nor indeed anyone or indeed any entity involved in the chain of supply resulting in your current reading experience, can or will be held legally responsible for anything untoward happening to your person as a result of your experimentation based on information presented herein. By the same token we do not expect credit for any positive results either. This is your book now, and your trip (in other words), and so your responsibility.

Thank you.

Barefoot Doctor, London 2001

INDUCTION

There isn't much time, so I won't waste any attempting to flam you with nonsense. There's far too much of that around as it is and my self-given remit is to deliver valuable perception-changing information with the minimum of fuss or extraneous textual posturing.

The purpose of this opening item is to draw you in, to seduce you and to induce you to overcome, override or simply bypass any resistance you may have to allowing these words to penetrate your consciousness.

And that is a very cheeky thing to do.

I'm fully taking advantage of a time-honored illusion we still cherish – that the printed word is sacrosanct and that a whole pile of printed words shaped into the cubic mass of a book such as this is approximately sixty thousand times more so.

On the one hand it's true. By sucking this body of text into your circuits you will inevitably instigate a fundamental change in the way you perceive and experience reality – and for that this book may well be worthy of its sacred status. On this basis, the same can be said for a fast-food hamburger, which will, through its interaction with your gut, also set up a chain of chemical effects that will fundamentally alter your perception and experience. This is in fact the crux of what you are about to read – how your willingness to hold a hamburger sacred will lend your life meaning in the moment and, for a brief while, fill that irksome gap in your sense of wellbeing and integrity.

I'm saying this to immediately disinherit you of any false conceptions about this meeting (between you and I). I do so to free us both from unnecessary expectations. That way the process will be much more fun. I say process because gaining access to the most intimate part of your mind and introducing a whole raft of new concepts requires a process of you deciding to trust me enough to allow yourself to entertain the ideas I present for long enough to benefit materially from the substance thereof. Or at least to confuse you into a semi-trance state with long convoluted sentences (like the last one) or just by talking kinda funny as I tend to do – but why not if you can get away with it? (Hell, I'm a funny guy.)

Notice that I've started to wax personal rather early on in this dialogue, which you may consider impertinent, but surely there's enough charade going on in the world without me adding to it. I've always had little patience for the longwinded and awkward tangos danced in society to ease the transition from bullshit to authenticity. I tend to go straight in and connect eye to eye, mind to mind, heart to heart, soul to soul, spirit to spirit even. I can't be bothered to waste the time otherwise. Can you?

So I'm assuming an intimacy with you that you may not want to entertain. Furthermore, I'm doing so to induce you to experiment with a parcel of pragmatic existentialism, which though dating back in origin at least four thousand years still remains a highly volatile agent that can wreak havoc with the structure of your life. If you like things as they are and would like them to remain so, stop reading this now. However, if you happen to be an addict for high-speed transformation of both reality and the way you experience it – come what may – then read on (because you're gonna love it).

Experimenting with psychophysical techniques and the Taoist philosophy that spawned them, presented here by someone with decidedly wayward tendencies, may give rise to a period of unsettled emotions and disturbed mind states. In time, however, what occurs through this exchange will provide you with another useful 'substance' to stick in your personal medicine chest and use or abuse as you see fit.

You've been warned, now listen but decide for yourself.

What I want to talk about is the optimization of the remainder of your time here on Earth.

But before I do, it's only fair I clue you into the fact that I'm not God –not even one of the lesser angels – and though I may have found the magic key to the sacred realm of publishing and publicity, I am merely another flawed mortal just like you. Not more than human, but perhaps more human than some, I am consistently astounded by the juxtaposition presented by the depth of my knowledge and the dysfunctionality of my person. I am in fact (as I suspect you may be yourself) a mass of heaving contradictions and anomalies. Yes I do hold the keys to enlightenment and yes I do use them to open my doors of perception with frequency and regularity and to teach or help others to do so too. But in the business of teaching and helping I am also very much living in this world and, like you, wish to guzzle all its fruits till satiated.

With over thirty years of religiously practicing Taoist and other self-realization methods, I've managed to find a way that helps me to guzzle with relatively little indigestion. It is a way that is discreet, rarely gives cause for embarrassment, fits with any dress code and yet still makes for interesting dinner-party conversation.

In fact, it's a way you already know instinctively – the Tao means the natural way after all. My job as teacher here is merely to remind you of a 'space' you've been aware of since you were very young, by speaking to that part of you that already resonates with the Tao, whether you knew it or not. And if that's all I manage here, to remind you in my weird and witty way of your own personal Tao, then I shall be content – we can never be reminded enough, as any Buddha or barefoot doctor will tell you.

I've actually practiced everything in this book on myself every day for nearly thirty years – not because of any misguided sense of spiritual obedience or Virgoan goody-goodiness, but because if I didn't 'do' my two hours a day, I'd probably seize up and go completely nuts. So though I can't validly proclaim this way of the Doctor is good for everyone, I can say without reservation that it's damn good for me and if it works for a madman like me, it can probably work for you too.

Anyway, enough of me. This is your book now, not mine, so without further ado, let me morph into servant mode and proceed to present you with a slew of data that is guaranteed to rip your psychic underwear off with its teeth.

However, in case you fall prey to the superficial allures of the warrior ethic, it should be stated that (as any accomplished martial artist will tell you) no matter your manner or style of external interaction, no matter the fashions or trends you subscribe to, no matter your choice of hairstyle and no matter whether you go barefoot or not, the real business of being a warrior takes place internally. When all your internal forces are in harmony, your external conditions, including all your interactions with other people and objects, hairstyles and so on, will reflect that harmony instantaneously or shortly thereafter and you will find yourself walking your warrior talk in ever fresher pastures.

I will mention the 'Tao': a word or sound meaning the undifferentiated absolute or, in common parlance, God, where both existence and non-existence originate, and as 'Him', 'Her' or however you prefer it, sparingly, as it's still a dirty word or sound for some, implying as it does an affinity with old-school religions that have harmed (as well as helped) many in the past. When I do, be assured that I only refer to 'God' in the transpersonal, unpersonified form, unaffiliated to any religion, as that which is the assumed ontological ground for both existence (in this case yang) and non-existence (in this case yin), the 'Tao' in other words.

Which is all well and good, but how does it benefit you and how do you roll it out into the marketplace?

At the root of everything about to be imparted is learning the ability to return voluntarily on a regular basis to that deepest level of reality – the Tao – as if it were a rejuvenating spiritually scented bubble bath. The Taoists of the ancient Orient (and I say 'Orient' and not 'China' because Taoism spread and was developed throughout the entire region under different guises, hence the Japanese suffix 'do' – Tao – attached to judo and aikido for example) discovered that such returning would imbue them with a 'supernatural' power, which beneficially affected them on all levels of being, from the spiritual through the physical to the profane. They called this power 'chi', and found that learning to develop and circulate it throughout their bodies made them look and feel younger and sexier, increased their charisma, and helped them feel strong, relaxed and healthy. They also discovered that chi could be used for self-defense and healing and thus could help them deal more equanimously and graciously with others. They even found chi helped make ideas manifest – make dreams come true, in other words – partly because of their increased social agility but partly also because chi is an alchemical agent.

They also realized (as you may yourself if you experiment with this material) that the more you generate chi, or energy, from within, the less you need to siphon it off from other people, and therefore the less trouble you'll find yourself in in the long run. Not that a Taoist, ancient or modern, would say it's bad to share energy with each other. On the contrary, sharing energy with others when all concerned are generating that energy from within is what moves mountains, or at least produces true social change and the possibility of peace and abundance. But they knew that until everyone was attuned to this approach, the chances of getting messed up increased the more people you had daily commerce with.

But as you might imagine, these characters had meditation time on their hands and easily affordable mountainside retreats to spend it in. There wasn't as much to do in those days – the listings magazines were all but empty. It was fine for them to sit for hours in meditation developing their connection to the Tao – source of the sauce, the chi. They didn't have to deal with the incessant bleeping of the 'William Tell Overture' on their mobile phones, or that running, mounting backlog of emails and text messages. They didn't have to keep up with the contents of five hundred TV channels to have an eye on the culture. They didn't care anyway. Can you imagine 14 million Taoists tuning into a daily soap?

But what about those mad devils caught in the mass particle accelerator of post-modern life (you and I)? How could you (or I) possibly benefit from something as arcane and apparently time-consuming as returning to the source when we already have such over-brimming schedules?

In fact, sessions of entering the Tao occur in a dimension beyond time as we usually know it. It takes less than a minor portion of a nanosecond to slip through the gap, and if you're really practiced it only takes the same to regenerate your chi for many hours or more. And if you're really-really practiced you learn to maintain awareness of both realities simultaneously. Beyond that stage is the awareness that there is only the Tao, or however you wish to refer to it, and all else is mere scenic decoration. You may think you'd have to be extremely enlightened to achieve such a state, but all you need to be is awake. The only quality the Buddha would admit to possessing, by the way, was awakeness – he reckoned that was all you needed to free yourself from suffering.

All the 'high-speed spirituality' methods in this book, comprising some of the most hardcore Taoist awakening practices known to humans, can be practiced at breakneck tempo and will fit comfortably into those micro-moments of downtime that crop up between breaths in the process of an intensely busy urban day.

I'm not about to glorify it, don't worry – we all know the city is a huge, filthy dump – but it's addictive. So addictive that, rather than have the sense to leave it alone, we've managed to spread it across the face of the globe – poetically just in time for the sea to wash it all away. This notwithstanding (and it's a big notwithstanding), the image of the global city works best if you consider the still 'wild' bits as theme parks and the urban hubs as the global equivalent of yesterday's local high streets. In other words, however far you go, you'll always more or less loosely be caught within the urban net.

This is not written plaintively: global urbanization is merely a result of the organic process of humans peopling the planet, we must assume, and not an aberration of nature, as some would have us believe. For no matter how much you may blame technology for our troubles, none of it came from anywhere else than right here on the planet. And humans tend to people places by congregating, not generally by isolating themselves. And we will congregate with the help of any medium we can lay our hands on whether virtual or real. This is because we have to. We cannot survive without each other's help. And that's without getting romantic about it. We cannot survive without each other's attention, love, energy, warmth, ideas, labor or produce.

In short, we are severely addicted to one another and that is why we are addicted to the city (in the abstract, global context) – we crave (or are repelled by) its energy, which represents the synergistic sum of all our energies combined. We are energy junkies.

Paradoxically, as you know, this very survival mechanism (the congregating tendency) is also the mechanism by which we are destroying ourselves – and rather swiftly too it would seem.

The urban experience indeed offers energy in the form of unlimited possibilities: excitement, filth, noise, commerce, innovation, pressure, sex, speed, drugs, danger, opportunity, 24-hour supermarkets, adventure, claustrophobia, agoraphobia, freedom, entrapment, wealth, poverty, abundance, scarcity, sophistication, depravity, opulence, squalor, grandeur, decay, regeneration, anonymity, recognition, isolation, connectedness, more pressure, release, entertainment, distraction, brutal reality, hardcore fantasy, culture, base animal instincts, violence, lust, love, fear and loathing – often all at once – and all in the space of a couple of blocks.

Add or subtract from the list as you will, it's a heady mix whichever way you play it. And we do play it every way and everywhere possible, as a result of which, no matter your location as you read this, you are inevitably inextricably bound up to some degree in the proliferation of effects – positive and negative – of the global city.

Though you don't have to be in an urban hub to enjoy the global city's dubious delights – you could be at a cyber or real-time satellite site situated in one of the world's great tourist theme parks, Thailand, Peru, up the Rocky Mountains or even the English countryside for instance – obviously the nearer to a hub you are, the stronger the intensity of experience. (Intensity of experience is an intrinsic part of the energy addiction – as an addict you need more energy and you need it delivered more intensively as time goes by.)

You are as vulnerable to the dangers of this energy as you are available to receive its benefits. It can kill you as easily as it can heal you. Right now, collectively speaking, the signs are it's killing us. The addiction is finally taking its toll. But maybe we can tip the balance by going to the source for our energy instead of to each other. If, by degrees, we learn to feed ourselves energetically from within more, we will need to rely less on the energy output of others in all its myriad forms, the interchange of which is currently pulling too heavily on the planet's resources to allow our species' survival.

The implication of this is that you are presented every moment, this one for instance, with a choice.

Do you interface as a victim tossed helpless in the winds of mounting chaos, violence, disease, global insanity (especially at leadership level) and ecological meltdown, or do you interface as a warrior?

A WARRIOR!

While there is something quaint about using the warrior archetype as your template for successful living, there is no doubt of its instant appeal. Think samurai, think Cain in 'Kung Fu', think ninja, think Carlos Casteneda's Don Juan, Ghengis Khan, Boadicea, even think El Cid. Now preface it with 'urban' (the magic filthy word) – urban warrior – and all sense of the quaint dissolves instantly to reveal a new post-modern archetype of equal relevance and use to both sexes.

The urban warrior metaphor implies the traditional warrior qualities – discipline, compassion, spiritual awakeness, perceptiveness, humility, modesty, clarity, tolerance, forgiveness, humor, cheerfulness, authenticity (integrity or virtue), dignity, grace or graciousness, strength or fortitude, tenacity, courage (to risk all), wisdom, kindness, sensitivity, naturalness, composure, confidence, charisma, sex-appeal, hygiene, diplomacy, tact, peacefulness, kindness, love, protection, and originality – all this but with a post-modern twist, mixed with good dress sense of course.

But why warrior? Are we at war? Yes. With ourselves, each other, our environment and with the force of nature that generates us itself. If your curiosity is aroused, rendering you desirous of some rather nifty detail to help you optimize your chances of winning this war, don't hang about. Keep reading, keep reading.

HIGH SPEED

As with any addiction, your craving for energy obtained through interaction with others increases the more you take. The proliferation of media through which interaction can take place exponentially increases both the volume and frequency of interactivity, raising tolerance levels and fueling greater craving. You want more and you want it now. The recent quantum leap in the speed of communication may well soon be counterbalanced by a brief anti-technology backlash, possibly abetted by a global economic downturn. But this is likely only to serve to ease the accelerator pedal off the floor and steady it somewhere still way above the legal speed limit. In this super-fast-tempo interactivity milieu we've grown used to, the most realistic hope for survival, short-term at least, is a naturally evolved high-speed cruise control.

For short of catastrophic developments like asteroidal collision impact, large-scale landmass flooding, global war using weapons of mass destruction, utter food chain breakdown, raging global plague epidemics, irreversible environmental damage, total global economic collapse, governmental ineptitude or socio-civic unrest reaching uncontrollable proportions, there is nothing that will induce us to voluntarily put a foot, bare or otherwise, on the brakes – except maybe Interactivity Speed Freaks Anonymous (ISFA), which doesn't exist yet, but look out for it, it's bound to spring up soon.

Fact is, as you know, all the above examples of factors that would contribute to a sudden let up in pace are alarmingly far from far-fetched. But the game's not over yet and while there's life there's hope. While there's hope, there's excitement, and while there's excitement, there's high-speed interactivity, even though it's this very speed that's increasing the probability of all the above examples (even the asteroids, if you look from a metaphysical standpoint).

Unlike other self-help, stress-reduction teachings, however, I in no way advocate slowing down your interactivity rate –this would be to go against the flow of the Tao or nature. On the contrary, speed up and increase the frequency and volume of interaction till your eyes spin in their sockets and your brain explodes through the top of your head, if you find it fulfilling. Meantime, use it to trigger your enlightenment. Or what's the point?

SPIRITUALITY (OTHERWISE WHAT'S THE POINT!)

When I was 19 or so, an elderly Tibetan lama looked with great compassion into my eyes and said, 'Without thpirituality you are thimply wathting your time.' (He had a fetching lisp.) Glancing at his robes arranged neatly about his cross-legged form and his beatific smile redolent of his seventy-odd years spent in inward-gazing austerity at the monastery, I promptly replied, 'I know you're right, but I've got things to do in the world first. I'll get into the spirituality later when I'm done.' He simply chuckled in response.

It's OK, I'm not about to launch into one of those faux-new age tales of how I then went off to the high-mountain deserts and spent time finding myself, in the bizarre company of a Native American shaman – though strangely I did – or even how I was once captured by a tribe of frenzied can-can dancers on the French Riviera. However, through my subsequent studies of Taoism and other self-help ways, it became obvious over the years that it's not a question of the spiritual or the profane, but the spiritual and the profane. In this multiple-choice, multiple-orgasm world of ours, it would be cruel to deny yourself or others the freedom to experience and possibly enjoy guzzling all the fruits on offer. After all, how much fruit can a person eat? However, if you were to do so in your sleep, without spiritual awareness in other words, you'd be missing the very gist of the action and what would be the point? The Tibetan was right, without spiritual awareness – without being awake like the Buddha – you'd be simply wasting your precious time here.

Why!

Let me pin down a definition of 'spirituality' here and now, which will hopefully both serve to explain why, as well as to put something down for posterity before this already over-used word comes to be nothing more than a synonym for a packet of joss-sticks.

Spirituality, the practice of noticing the presence of spirit, is a natural faculty, well known to small children up to the age of 8, before conventional schooling has taken its toll, and there-after usually not until the first flush of puberty-driven sexual activity has calmed down at, say, 18 or whenever you first get your heart properly broken, your romantic delusions about life shattered, and feel a compelling need to do something about your existential pain.

The difference between these stages is that small children move naturally and spontaneously in and out of the 'practice', often unconsciously, but as an adult, the only way in is by conscious choice. This choice involves a decision to override habitual thought patterns acquired during the school years, to momentarily defuse the power of the rational, judgmental or cynical mind and surrender or slip into the silence of the great existential void within. This runs counter to the general trend, which is to avoid the void at all costs by losing oneself in the distraction of interaction (with others, directly or indirectly).

You dread the silence of the void as if it were death itself (with which it is synonymous), fearing that if you were to pause for one moment, horror would rush in to fill the gap. But as any young child or member of any ancient pre-consumerist society will tell you, the existential void, with all its implications of death, is in fact your very best friend in the world.

Surely you had those experiences as a child where you'd hear the voices of friendly invisibles giving counsel in your inner ear? Or you'd find yourself in a spontaneous state of polydimensional unity and empathy with your surroundings and sometimes even get a sense of the ubiquity of benign consciousness throughout all time and space and your intrinsic pro-active connection with it all? Surely there were times you knew with all your heart, soul and mind that your prayers were being heard and instantaneously acted upon by a force you'd have been quite happy calling 'Tao', if only because it was less of a mouthful than 'Thomas the Tank Engine'? Surely there were moments you remember touching or being touched by sudden unexpected acts of human kindness and almost visibly seeing the grace subsequently released into the surrounding atmosphere? Surely you have a catalogue of instances when your heart's deepest wish was made manifest before your very eyes, the process of which gave you the undeniable sensation of a benign invisible presence, neither somewhere within you nor somewhere outside of you, but both? Surely you remember praying for help in aeroplanes on meeting with major turbulence on a night-flight over say the North Atlantic and saying 'thank you' when you landed?

It's OK, I've finished 'surelying' you now. I was only using it as a hypnotic device (repetition of stimulus to numb the local mind) to stop you thinking habitually and instead feel into that spiritual space within and surrounding you, which is after all entirely natural and familiar to you. Without feeling, it's all just so many words and – with spirit being indescribable – wasted words at that.

But I'm not about to suggest that all you have to do is find your confounded inner child and converse with the fairies to become an enlightened post-modern master (or mistress), though of course you can if that's how you swing. In fact, learning to be able to slip into the spiritual space at will requires more than a degree of self-discipline and application – you'll have to be a warrior about it, and I don't mean in the manner of a toy soldier or even a Christian one for that matter.

You'll have to be a warrior in the sense of remaining awake and alert even while you sleep, like a soldier in the midst of battle. Whatever form of interaction you're engaged in, whether with a person or group of people, for social, economic or sexual commerce (offline or on), whether with an object (a steering wheel for instance), whether with your own internal fantasies and projections, you train yourself to remember to stay mindful of the presence of spirit.

It's like remaining aware that you're in a cinema while watching the movie and therefore not getting so lost in the cinematic action that your life falls apart when the closing credits start scrolling up on the screen. It's like framing your experience of local reality in a far broader context, a limitless context in fact, which you can broaden according to your current whim and capacity. The broader the context of experience, the greater the view. The greater the view the more information, hence wisdom, is yours. The greater your wisdom, the wiser your moment-to-moment choices will become. The wiser your moment-to-moment choices become, the more easily and adroitly you'll negotiate your way through the apparent maze of life on Earth in the global city till it's time to get off the planet. Moreover, when you finally do leave you will have the opportunity of doing so with fear at a minimum and clarity at a maximum. You will have seen through the illusion of death (and life), thus being more free in the final moment to fully appreciate and enjoy what surely must be the most profound and important experience of all: popping your clogs.

So that's spirituality. It has nothing to do with joss-sticks, though if you choose wisely they do help the room smell nicer and can cover up a whole host of airborne sins (the horrible perfume of a guest, tobacco smoke or worse), which in turn can be pleasing to the spirits, as they say in India. But they also act as a smokescreen, so let's move on.

PEOPLE ON THE RUN

You run from death, you run from the existential void, you run from your fear, your sadness, your grief and your anger. You run from the past. You run from the future. Mostly you run from the present. You run from others. You run from the fact of being on a relatively small and unlikely planet – your only viable life-raft for many light years around, moving at 19 miles per second through deep, dark, cold, airless, endless space vulnerable to a local (yet omnipotent) and increasingly volatile weather system. You run from the underlying truth beneath all your suppressed or overt feelings of isolation and alienation, namely that you enter this game alone and leave it thus, this being true no matter how popular, successful, powerful, sexy, enlightened or even how well dressed you are.

You run because, in all this distraction, you get excited. You run because the game's damn fast and if you don't keep up you don't survive. You run because with the way things are going in mass transit, it could be the quickest way to get to work. You run because you love it and travelling at 19 miles per second is just too slow not to try and improve upon.

It's become fashionable to be on the run. Who's got time to walk or dawdle, unless on a specified walking- or dawdling-to-ease-inner-stress vacation? It makes you feel romantic about your life, like a post-modern outlaw or double-time gypsy.

So run.

But in your running you have a choice. You can run like a warrior (in battle) or you can run like a headless chicken (the way of shopping and fucking).

In fact, running like a warrior is part of Taoist training – its called 'flying on land', and will be discussed in the book, training in which itself is used as a somatic metaphor for handling life in the fast lane with equipoise. Running like a warrior, in other words, has always been a respected notion.

A practiced runner knows breath control, pacing, direction setting, perseverance, co-ordination, relaxation in movement and when to stop and rest.

A practiced outlaw, as in one who is on the run, knows how not to get snagged in the wrong story lines that could result in permanent entrapment, and how to move through town without making traces.

The running outlaw, the urban warrior – you get the picture (before we both tangle ourselves in my metaphors).

A headless chicken running, on the other hand, knows nothing but running in pointless circles between one bout of consuming and consummating (shopping and fucking) and the next.

So assuming you're with me, more or less, on the 'flying on land' option, consider the idea of being constantly and consistently plugged into the unmovable Tao while negotiating your way through the external manifestations of the Tao, the '10 thousand things', at high speed. And this affording you absolute clarity, limitless energy and an unshakeable sense of wellbeing no matter what. Because this is exactly what is up for consideration in the next section of text.

Every session of hypnosis – for after all is that not what we do with each other, engage in mutual hypnosis? – begins with an induction to trip up the local, subjective 'layer' of mind and thus gain access to a deeper 'layer' way beneath the surface where all the real, as opposed to ideal, choices are made. For ultimately, it's choice we are concerned with here. The choice whether or not to be a headless-chicken-syndrome victim or a warrior flying gracefully and purposefully on land; whether to remain asleep or to wake up; whether to make the least or the most of your remaining time here on Earth; and whether or not it really is OK to wear brown shoes with navy slacks.

When the hypnotherapist has come to the end of his or her induction routine and has finally finished playing childishly with you in the above fashion, he or she then proceeds to escort you down to that deeper stratum of choice-making consciousness, known to practitioners of shamanism as 'the underworld'.

Hopefully you will have arrived at that stage, enabling me to converse directly with that deeper layer of your mind, in order to impart in full depth the Taoist outlook and philosophy. Knowledge of this is fairly prerequisite to your full appreciation of the actual methods contained later in the book – knowledge that could be wasted in the harsh, cold light of day if addressed solely to your local, subjective, workaday self.

POSITIVE POLYPHRENIA

Inside you are countless selves. Amongst whom there's the decent one, the indecent one, the honest, virtuous one, the lying, thieving one, the loving, generous one, the hateful, mean one, the wise, peaceful one, the stupid, violent one, the secure one, the insecure one, the sexy, confident one, the frumpy, shy one, the sly, deceitful one, the open, honorable one, the feminine one, the masculine one, the old one, the young one, the bold one, the timid one, the crazy, drunken one, the sane, sober one, the materially inclined one, the spiritually inclined one and so on (and on).

Pulling that rabble into enough of an order to get through the day in a relatively straight line is a great feat of self-organization requiring strong internal leadership qualities. Those who do not naturally possess these qualities may be fortunate enough to learn them on the run. Or they could end up identifying with one or more selves and getting stuck in a behavioral loop, which at best severely limits their experiential scope and at worst lands them in an institution or pushes them to commit violent crimes. (Institution here can of course refer to the institution of national government as much as to the insane asylum – government leaders and players are not unknown to display symptoms of pathological polyphrenic loop syndrome, which is exactly what causes wars.)

For the sake of argument, let's call this syndrome negative polyphrenia and its opposite positive polyphrenia. Polyphrenia, by the way, means many-minded, as opposed to schizophrenia, which actually means a mind split in two by a schism. Poly does not imply a schism, it merely means the many.

So here you are, expected to preside over the internal multitude, to lead them wisely as a cohesive unit through the obstacles and pitfalls of the high-resolution graphic computer game of post-modern urban life, but who exactly are you? Who actually does the leading?

The one who leads is the one who experienced weightlessness in the womb, who felt constriction passing through the birth canal, who woke up terrified from a childhood nightmare, who experienced the pain of falling over and the triumph of winning a race, who witnessed the ageing process in the bathroom mirror but never felt any older, who knew the bliss of love, who suffered the pain of loss and was blessed by the mercy of sleep, who was filled with awe on seeing the heights of the mountains and the vastness of the night sky, who cried with joy at the birth of a child, who pierced the veil and slipped through to the other side at the end of the ride and who still didn't feel any older, who also got absolutely out of it the other night to the point of amnesia – it's that which forgot, that's who leads. (Which is why a true warrior never gets so drunk or otherwise as to become internally leaderless – because in the ensuing political vacuum, you never know which self among the many will take command. The chances are, as you know from experience, it will be one of the rogues and we all know what happens then.)

Now imagine yourself the leader, standing on the balcony of the presidential pile, gazing down at the crowd gathered in the presidential plaza below. The sound of a thousand selves each voicing their individual fears and longings fills your ears. You do not react. You simply listen. You relax. The palace gates are well guarded – you can afford to be benevolent. You assimilate and consider all the various conflicting demands of the crowd below, make a decision and issue the command.

The rabble are happy to subordinate themselves to your will because you're a kind, wise and loving leader. They know you'd please all of them if you could, but you can't so you won't. And they accept that because you, the 'one', are strong. It's a benign dictatorship. An internal democracy is unworkable – it's what leads to walking round the streets talking aloud to people who aren't actually there. And a malevolent dictatorship! Well you can try but it'll cause you stress, as anyone who has spent their life beating themselves up will tell you.

This 'one', this benign dictator, represents your spirit, which, when properly situated and comfortably settled within, will lead your polyphrenic being through life in accordance with your true nature – not pretending or denying in other words – to bring you optimum value and pleasure from every remaining moment.

It does not use force in order to achieve this. Instead it leads from behind, languishing all the while in the spiritual bubble bath. It assimilates and considers all the fears and longings expressed by the many within and issues the appropriate command to facilitate a feasible compromise for all involved.

Thus you are led by your spirit within and in accord with the flow of the Tao.

Which is a fine concept if you can follow it, but how do you take it from the imaginary and make it happen in real time?

THROUGH THE BODY

'Your body is your temple, but it's also your nightclub' Raja Ram.

Religion, repetitiously reading the Holy Scripture, following the word in other words, requires faith. Following scripture written in the distant past by other humans, whether you believe in its heavenly origins or not, implies being led by a divine force external to you. A benign deity beyond the stained glass window where all the spiritual action goes on. Which is fine as long as you feel more comfortable with the illusion of being once removed from the spiritual realm, separated by priests and doctrine from the full fury and glory of the Tao.

Taoism, on the other hand, is the practice of pragmatic existentialism and requires no acts of blind faith. Taoism is a word used to describe the practice of various psychophysical techniques designed to afford you direct access to the spiritual realm whence derives the warrior's power – a backstage pass, access all areas, in other words.

You're not just kneeling down and standing up and singing songs to it, you are it.

However, this in no way implies a choice to be made between religion and Taoism – that would be about as meaningful as a choice between, say, eating or sitting down. You can do both at once if you want. But it does mean that if you happen to be unencumbered by the baggage of religion or superstition yet value the importance of the spiritual connection, there is a suck-it-and-see method of attaining it, here and now on the spot (if you want it).

And the way you do it is through the body. You no longer need ritual, dogma or church buildings to gain access to the spiritual realm.

Your body is the temple in the sense of being your point of entry into the Tao.

The 'one' in you who leads the internal rabble is comfortably settled and optimally poised only when properly situated. And that proper situation is within the body – specifically located within an internal somatic architecture so eloquently expressed in the Taoist model.

There's a time and a place for everything these days, which is why your body is not only a temple but a nightclub too. As well as being your access point to the spiritual realm, your body is also your point of access to the realm of the pleasures of the flesh. And it's crucial that this realm is not denied or suppressed, for to do so is to constrict the very spirit you are trying to reach to and will give rise to grave disharmony.

These two, the ethereal and temporal, spirit and matter, are in fact inseparable, at least within your body. In Taoism, as with the animistic spiritual ways of the Native Americans who also originally hailed from Asia, spirit is not superior to matter but coexists with it on the same level. Spirit is a force or dimension to be played with and enjoyed rather than revered or feared.

Thus is one able to experience a shopping or fucking expedition as a spiritual event, seeing the sales assistant or lover as personifications of the divine and the objects purchased as animated with spirit or the orgasm an expression of spiritual bliss.

Thus is one able to indulge in pleasures of the senses enhanced perhaps by drugs or alcohol and still remain in a state of spiritual purity.

In fact, purity has little to do with the high toxicity of what you ingest and much to do with the low toxicity of your thoughts, especially when concerning others.

Spiritual and profane – it all transpires within your body.

And the linking mechanism?

YOUR BREATH

Other than its obvious crucial importance to both your immediate and longer-term survival, your breathing mechanism provides the primary linking device to unity spirit and local self.

This device can only be employed effectively, however, when the breath is allowed and encouraged to flow freely both during its ingress and egress. To achieve this you don't have to do anything new, you have to stop doing something old: holding your breath.

Holding your breath occurs unconsciously more often in a day than you'd care to imagine as a reflex contraction of the diaphragm – the horizontally placed muscle in the upper abdominal region that controls the bellows-like motion of the lungs – as a defense against stress. It happens after breathing in and just before breathing out. Breathing in fills your thoracic cavity. Retaining the breath creates the illusion of being substantial in the face of the perceived tidal wave of life-pressure. However, all it does is exacerbate stress by causing constriction of the thoracic musculature, thus blocking blood and energy circulation. Furthermore, when holding the breath like this, the ensuing exhalation is rarely a full one, which hinders the lungs' ability to cast out toxins. This in turn places strain on both kidneys and liver, which in turn causes, among other things, grouchiness and down-heartedness.

The first step to spiritual enlightenment, then, is training yourself to stop holding your breath, except of course when swimming considerable distances underwater without breathing equipment.

You can help yourself remember by placing a free palm on your upper abdomen at regular intervals throughout the day and night, especially while engaged in conversation with others, whether face to face or on the phone, and during stressful moments.

The second step is to train yourself to slow the breath down. Consciously decelerating your breathing tempo is one of the most powerful self-regulatory tools at your disposal. It's the only way you can pace your energy flow, calm your mind when it gets anxious, restless or confused and even decrease your pulse rate when required. The way to train yourself into this habit is to consciously extend your out breath to the count of, say, nine and consciously do the same with the in breath. Complete nine cycles of this in a row, once a day for nine days, and it'll start to occur naturally of itself.

As any great composer, conductor or dancer will tell you, tempo is a key factor in the organization of a piece of music, unless of course it is intentionally arrhythmic. So it is for the dance of daily life, where sensitivity to both your internal tempo and the external tempo of local events is crucial to the appropriate timing of your words and actions. By decelerating your breath tempo you internally hook onto an easy half-time groove that will enable you to remain relaxed in the midst of high-speed action. Moreover, if you are a subscriber to the Oriental belief that you're born with a pre-allocated number of breaths to last you this life-time, the final one of which means death, it would make sound sense to slow the process down as much as you can if you're at all interested in personal life span extension.

This is all well and good, but if you don't have a proper handle on the correct mechanics of the breathing action itself, the whole process will become rather too much of a chesty, top- heavy affair to afford you full benefit.

To make full use of your lungs, which after all is free – and to do otherwise would be like only choosing fifty grand if I offered you a hundred for nothing – you have to reverse the normal Western pattern to the effect that when you inhale, your entire belly expands, while when you exhale, your belly contracts. Throughout, your chest remains relatively still.

To help you visualize this, picture a large sea-sponge in your lower abdomen. Unlike a normal sponge, however, this one soaks up air instead of water. As you know, to get a sponge to suck in effectively it is always best to squeeze it out first.

Imagine, therefore, on exhalation contracting your abdominal muscles by consciously pulling them back towards your spine in order to compress the sponge and thus squeeze out the air. Now imagine the sponge filling with air of its own accord as you inhale.

Having visualized the process, try it in real-time while lying on your bed, or someone else's if you prefer, with a hand on your belly while completing nine full inhalation-exhalation cycles. Repeat this morning and night for nine days and it will start becoming habitual. (The significance of the number nine and other key numerals will be discussed later.)

In summary, stop holding your breath, slow your breathing down and breathe deeply, which as you now know does not mean noisily sucking air into your chest in the manner of someone about to inflate a child's balloon and blowing out in the manner of an orangutan in labor. On the contrary, with your breath flowing unimpeded and slowly in and out from your belly, not only will you encourage the mind state of a warrior, you will also help to prevent or cure constipation, IBS, high blood pressure, various circulatory and respiratory problems including asthma, anxiety, certain strains of insanity, premature ejaculation and even halitosis.

In fact, once this 'warrior Buddha' style of breathing becomes habitual, there will be very little that could knock you off balance in the course of a busy urban lifetime, especially when you combine this knowledge with the following (knowledge).

OPTIMUM ORGANIZATION OF ALL AVAILABLE FLESH AND BONES

To get maximum usage of the entire package, which is you, you have to relax. Nothing great is ever accomplished in a state of stress – any warrior will tell you that, urban or otherwise. Only when you're relaxed can your breath flow freely, your thoughts run in a meaningful sequence and your blood and energy circulate unobstructed. Relaxation is a physical phenomenon. If you relax your muscles you relax your mind and vice versa.

But relaxing your muscles while collapsing your form will do you little good. Your physical form is supported primarily by your skeleton, which is under direct command of your mind. With your thoughts alone, you can cause your entire structure to crumple or grow at will.

By simply visualizing your spine lengthening upwards and your shoulder and hipbones broadening outwards, your entire physical form will actually expand and grow.

Once your bones have been arranged to allow optimum expansion of the form, it is easy to relax the flesh, by simply visualizing it softening on the bone and sinking towards the ground, counter to the upward pull of the spine.

Hence the bones create the shape you want to make, whether in stillness or in motion, and the muscles, tendons and ligaments merely move the bones.

This saves you inordinate amounts of energy normally squandered on the muscular strain of holding the body together around a misaligned skeletal structure. Moreover, with the skeleton arranged to facilitate optimum expansion of form and the muscles working more effectively, the increased chi, or energy, in your system can flow freely bringing you the instant benefits of a healing and self-protective energetic 'sheath'.

All that and we're not even 10 thousand words into the book.

To translate these images into physical fact, however, you need to keep a vigilant eye from now on, on the way you lie, sit, stand, walk, run, skip, hop, jump, climb stairs, dance, copulate and get in and out of cars (especially if you're a celebrity subject to the paparazzi lens) – whether at work, rest or play. Remember as often as possible to check for full vertical and horizontal skeletal expansion with simultaneous softening and sinking of the muscles at all times. You may feel a need to practice this consciously while lying, sitting and standing still before taking it out on the road.

But as I say, you're still only 10 thousand words or approximately a quarter of a mile of text into the book. For further refinement, imbibe this ...

INTERNAL SOMATIC ARCHITECTURE

Let's, for the sake of argument, say that occupying the same space as your internal organs, bowels and brain is a subtle architecture, a metaphysical anatomy existing in the fifth dimension – the realm of spirit.

Invisible to the naked eye while looking outwards, it is revealed only when the gaze is turned inwards – as long as your gaze knows what to look out for, of course.

It consists of a trio of linked psychic chambers: one in the middle of your brain, one in the middle of your chest and one in the middle of your lower abdomen. They are known in Taoist cosmology as 'tan tiens', meaning, 'fields of heaven' – similar to the ancient Greek concept of the Elysian fields – psychic fields within the physical body through which the heavenly (spiritual) force or Tao is able to act locally upon and through your system.

They are connected to each other by an energy super-conduit known as the 'penetrating' channel, which is approximately 2 inches in diameter – or at least would be if it was a purely physical phenomenon – and runs from between your legs, up the front face of your backbone and into your brain.

The rear aspect of each chamber is 'attached' to the front face of the penetrating channel via a little back door to facilitate easy access.

Via this penetrating channel, these inner chambers are also connected to seven other super-conduits comprising an eight-channel energy meta-network running throughout the body. Their task is to introduce spiritual intelligence – universal consciousness in other words – into your body's local energy network with which it connects, itself consisting of twelve meridians, each responsible for a different organ or bowel, and overall responsible for your local day- to-day survival on the planet.

If your body is the hardware, the local energy network of twelve organ- or bowel-related meridians is the operating system. The meta-system of eight super-conduits and three psychic chambers is the program you install to be able to function on the planet as a fully realized spiritual being – a warrior empowered with full universal consciousness as you wander (hopefully) immune to danger and disease in the midst of local events, urban or otherwise – providing you know how to work the program. (The clear and concise instruction manual for which is about to unfold before your very eyes.)

MAKING FULL USE OF YOUR UPPER CHAMBER

Roughly in the region of your pineal gland, that eye-shaped protuberance in the center of your brain, whose purpose still largely remains a mystery to Western science, is what's referred to lovingly on the street as your 'cavity of original consciousness'.

If you take one thing home with you, other than remembering to breathe properly, take this.

Imagine a line intersecting your brain from front to back, starting at the bridge of your nose and ending at the base of the occipital bone at the back of your skull. And now a second line running between your ear holes and intersecting the first in the dead center of your brain, between and behind your eyes approximately 3 inches back.

You may want to spend a moment with your eyes closed locating it. As you do so, however, be aware that you are already engaging in esoteric practices that could change things forever and should desist immediately if wishing to avoid possible internal turbulence, which can occur at the initial stages of program activation.

On closing your eyes and locating this intersection, you will find yourself in a vast Tardis-like inner chamber – its dimensions unfettered by the width or height restrictions of its physical container (your head).

Position your awareness carefully at this intersection, face front, as it looking out from this point and let your gaze rest on the view of endless inner space provided on the (imaginary) screen on the back of the forehead in front of you.

From your vantage point here in the upper chamber you will be able to witness the dazzling display of thoughts – normally experienced as the incessant sound of internal chatter between your many selves – as so many computer generated shapes – phantasms of light and color dancing across the screen against its background pattern of endless (inner) space. Each thought arises out of the depths of nowhere and returns thence, as you sit securely and unmoveable in the midst of your upper chamber, simply enjoying the internal show of dancing shapes.

As you do so, waste no energy following any particular shape or stream of shapes – the thoughts, in other words. Simply witness their arisal and dispersal. Resist the urge to judge or get involved with the content of any thought. Just see the thought emerge from the nothingness at the edge of the screen, dance across your line of vision and disappear again into the nothingness at the screen's other edge. Be sure to notice the disappearance of the thought, however, to avoid becoming inadvertently distracted by its content.

While observing a procession of thoughts, always keep an eye on the background of endless inner space. (And remember to breathe, for it is linking the experience to your breathing that makes it a somatic reality and not just another pile of worthless intellectual theory.)

When you find yourself lost in a thought stream, waste no energy berating yourself. Simply reassemble yourself posturally to enable maximum vertical and horizontal expansion of physical frame, relax, sink, breathe, concentrate your awareness in the middle of your brain and let your gaze rest once again on the view of endless inner space on the screen in front of you.

While on the subject of physical frame expansion, by the way, it should be pointed out, for the sake of good spiritual manners if nothing else, that all self-exploratory enterprises are far more likely to succeed when the spine is lengthened and aligned and the hips and shoulders broadened to facilitate an open feeling in the chest, belly, hips and across the back. In other (far fewer) words, it helps to sit up, stand up or lie down straight when you meditate. Not that I really want to get into using the 'm' word in polite company, but I should tell you that when engaging in the above-mentioned practice, you are in fact meditating. You should know this, as the practice of meditation may run counter to your religious beliefs or drug-taking habits and if so should be stopped immediately.

In fact, this is a perfect point to stop reading if you want to avoid acquiring potentially dangerous knowledge about how to maintain a state of full meditation while simultaneously externally engaged in the midst of daily life.

Because once you've grown accustomed to presiding magisterially over all of endless inner space from your unassailable vantage point in the midst of your upper chamber, it's a simple matter to maintain this vantage point with your eyes open whilst interacting with the world around you.

All you have to do is open your eyes.

However, as you do so, be sure to keep yourself 'sitting' comfortably at the central brain intersection within the safety of your upper chamber, gazing outwards through the portals provided by your (open) eyes.

Now the internal imagery of dancing thought-shapes is replaced by the external imagery of people and places – and of your interaction with them – dancing or rather acting before you in the drama of your everyday life. But you, the 'one', are still in the center of your brain.

So there you are. All those years devoting inordinate amounts of energy, time, worry and money on how you looked, when how you looked may well have been more a matter of how you look, as opposed to how you look, if you see what I'm getting at.

But that's not all there is to it.

An upper chamber cannot exist in isolation for long in a universe that depends, for the proper functioning of its external aspect at least, on the interrelated activity of all its parts. No, an upper chamber on its own will soon shrivel, die and fall out of the sky unless also firmly subtended by properly activated middle and lower chambers.

For this reason, let us, while leaving just enough awareness in the upper chamber to maintain a diplomatic presence there, cause our attention to descend swiftly down the slope (through the penetrating channel) to the middle chamber below.

An internal world built exclusively of an upper chamber without foundations is a top-heavy place, for sure, and one that is bound to topple – for a project to have legs it has to have heart too. And that's why it's imperative for your awareness to simultaneously reside in the middle chamber located approximately 5 inches back behind the center of your breastbone.

While your upper chamber is the proper situation for that aspect of the 'one' (in you) that watches, the middle chamber is the proper place for that aspect of the 'one' that feels. For without feeling (both pleasure and pain), imagine what a monotonously dull experience of existence you would have.

I won't go into a whole series of faux new-age blandishments about the importance of feelings and emotional intelligence – it's obvious that when your experience is wholly intellectual and without passion you become a dried-up old fish whom no one wants to talk to, not even you.

I won't try to sell you the idea of opening your heart, taking occupancy of your middle chamber in other words, by impressing on you how important it is to love (yourself, others and the world). Everyone knows that when you don't exercise your ability to love (energetically or physically express kind feelings towards self or others), you soon become the most unpopular boy or girl in the playground.

Anyone with a modicum of sensibility knows that without love and kindness any inner self-development work you do is just so much intellectual conceit and that a life – spiritually dedicated or otherwise – without passion, is a life wasted.

With that in mind, if you were to let your awareness rest a while in the middle chamber, 5 inches or thereabouts behind the center of your breastbone, you would no doubt find it a chamber of rare warmth and bonhomie, a most agreeable place, whose welcome was so comforting you'd never wish to leave again.

However, a man or woman has to do what a man or woman has to do and, as you know, that involves acting like a bit of an unloving arsehole from time to time. So be it. But if you can just maintain a small and humble presence there at all times, it will keep the saintly fires burning in your eyes enough to light your way through the darkness.

So, while observing your world from the upper chamber, allow yourself to feel it from the middle chamber, enjoying the warmth and expansiveness that radiates outwards from the front face of your spine at chest level as soon as you focus on it doing so. This is what gives your moment to moment experience its meaning. Always let your experience be supported by the warmth of your middle chamber.

If the upper chamber is where divine intelligence is sourced, the internally limitless proportions of your middle chamber house the source of your divine wisdom.

Or, put another way, keep your chest relaxed at all times while meditating.

Even so, a floating middle-and-upper-chamber complex, unsupported by a lower chamber, is even more likely to topple over than the simple floating single-chamber construction previously described. When you experience life only from these two chambers to the exclusion of the third, lower chamber, in other words, you are highly susceptible to raging delusions and subsequent faulty maneuverings through daily street life.

For the totality of your warrior self to be realized within, you must, leaving just enough awareness behind in the upper chamber to remain observant and sufficient in the middle chamber to remain emotionally responsive, descend to the very bowels of the Earth, so to speak –into the primal fire of the lower chamber itself.

HEAVEN AND HELL - THE LOWER CHAMBER

There is no doubt that our primitive superstitious belief in the eternal flames of hell owes its origins in the group psyche to a misinformed understanding of the power of the lower chamber.

While the eternal flames image is helpful, the eternal damnation associations are not.

In fact, it is crucial for overall harmony of the system, internally and in interaction with the external world, that the fire of the lower chamber is harnessed to support the middle and upper chamber. Unless, that is, you want to spend the rest of your time on the planet in a mere intellectually impassioned daydream.

The lower chamber is located approximately 6 inches behind a point itself located approximately 2 inches below your navel – bang in the middle of your lower abdomen and is not known in ancient Taoist circles as the 'Ocean of Limitless Energy' (chi) for nothing. Except that rather than being filled with salt-water, fish and other monsters, it's filled with the generative fire of life itself.

This is the fire that fuels your will – the will to move forward (backwards, sideways, up, down, in or out, as it were) from moment to moment. It is the fire that generates the energy that provides the warmth in the middle chamber and keeps the light bright in the upper chamber.

And it is, as you may have surmised, the same fire that fuels the base primal (survival) urges – creation and destruction – sex and violence. And it is on account of this function of course that there exists in the collective unconscious that association of the lower chamber, loins in other words, with the eternal flames of hell.

Indeed, without a sensible conscious presence simultaneously maintained in the middle and upper chambers (being in other words without wisdom and intelligence) activating the lower chamber to the exclusion of the other two will turn you into a craven, shagging, murdering maniac – or worse. Because conversely it is on account of a preponderance of energy unnaturally damned up in the lower body that the urge to commit violence or indulge in excessive promiscuity is given issue.

This is precisely why you must remain observant and awake in the upper chamber and open and emotionally responsive in the middle, whilst simultaneously making the potentially perilous descent into the fire of the lower chamber, if you wish to fan the flames of eternal life rather than those of damnation.

With this in mind, on allowing your awareness to settle in the lower abdomen, you will find the presence of a great force – or at least you will with practice. This is the power of life itself, the primal generative force capable of initiating new life, which instead you are harnessing to generate enough 'electricity' (chi) to warm and light up your entire internal kingdom or queendom.

The upper chamber houses that aspect of your 'one' that witnesses, the middle chamber houses that aspect that feels, the lower chamber houses that aspect that 'is' or that drives your 'isness'.

Experiment for a moment by closing your eyes and experiencing yourself situated simultaneously in all three chambers – watching existence from the upper chamber, feeling it in the middle chamber and driving it from the lower with equal presence. And remember to breathe (and relax).

I wouldn't suggest you practice this diligently for a few minutes on a daily basis with your eyes closed for approximately nine days so that it becomes automatic in order to be able to maintain it as an unshakeable inner experiential template even while engaged in the most distracting external events, unless you seriously see yourself as a proper urban warrior. If you're just into this for a brief bit of spiritual tourism and are planning to default to headless-chicken mode afterwards, it would in fact be better to forget the inflammatory nature of everything you've just read and stick to the basic not-holding-your-breath breathing advice. Otherwise, proceed with caution because it's time to start moving out through the meta network of eight energy super-conduits that regulate your universe to see what we can find. (Hold tight.)

EXPLORING THE SUPER-CONDUIT OF MAXIMUM UPWARD THRUST - STARTING WITH YOUR PERINEUM

Maintaining a viable conscious presence – a thought, in other words – in each of the three chambers, move out of the lower chamber downwards along the penetrating channel until you come to the perineum, that small area between your legs located directly in front of your anal opening and directly behind your genitals.

Your perineum is also known in Taoist circles as your 'gate of mortality' on account of its being an energetic valve, which when shut contains your chi (energy) thus preserving your assembled consciousness in the immortal or internally timeless state, but when open allows your energy to escape and thus your consciousness to dissipate (and die) externally in the world of the '10 thousand things'.

Even while reading, gently contract the muscles of your pelvic floor, squeezing and lifting the perineum upwards. Now re-expand the pelvic floor, allowing the perineum to relax and drop down again.

Conscious rhythmic perineal squeezing and relaxing is said to have been discovered by ancient Taoists who'd been observing the natural, habitual perineal motion of deer (though one is inclined to wonder at the degree of intimate exchange between Taoist and deer for such sensitive information to have been revealed).

That notwithstanding, it soon became clear to the deer-watching Taoists that such rhythmic perineal stimulation had a number of profound benefits. As well as helping to internally strengthen the prostate gland in men, thus helping prevent prostate cancer, and helping to internally strengthen the vaginal walls and uterus in women, thus helping to prevent uterine or ovarian cancer, rhythmically squeezing and releasing the perineum would increase one's sexual energy and one's ability to contain it at the same time. In other words, exercising the pelvic floor muscles (an activity normally only associated in polite Western society with pregnant women wishing to strengthen their vaginal walls and thus prevent post-partum muscle tone loss) fans the flames of the generative fire' in the lower chamber, while simultaneously increasing your ability to prevent it escaping unnecessarily through the gate of mortality' in pursuit of sexual (or consumerist) gratification.

Not that sexual gratification is wrong – far from it, and what a dried up old trout you'd soon become without it – but there is a trade off. The more you contain the fire in the lower chamber, thus enabling it to heat and light the middle and upper chambers, the more assembled, stable and satisfied in the moment will your spirit be and the more energy you'll have at your disposal, which is beneficial for longevity purposes. The more you allow the fire to escape through the gate on account of following a desire, the more your energy and spiritual integrity dissipates, which is not so beneficial for longevity purposes. But you can't live forever in this physical body, and who'd want to anyway – in such a crazy reality you need to read books like this to get by, so you trade off.

It's not only nice but also inevitable that you follow your desires from time to time. If you didn't there'd be no drama to live through and life would be a dull ride. With a complete absence of desire-following, after all, none of us would be here in the first place.

It's a question of balance. As long as you generally contain at least 51 per cent of the fire in the lower chamber you're in the black.

It's not a moral issue. The more you contain, the more you stabilize your warrior nature, the more you expend (shopping and fucking), the more you get lost in the world of headless chickens running round in circles. The choice is yours from moment to moment.

Meantime by rhythmically squeezing and releasing the perineum nine times, three times a day, starting now if you wish, you will instigate a pattern of containment. Moreover, your mental clarity will improve and your psychic awareness will increase.

Occasionally, try holding the squeeze at a comfortable level until you feel a pleasurable sensation of internal pressure pushing upwards through the penetrating channel into your lower chamber. Maintain the squeeze, feeling this sensation rise upwards along the channel to fill the middle chamber. Keep squeezing until the sensation is felt to rise through the channel to your upper chamber. Wait there squeezing for a moment, enjoying the gentle pressure in your brain, and then release the perineum and relax completely, allowing this sensation to drop back down the channel.

Throughout this 'operation', be sure to remember to remain aware and awake in the upper, middle and lower chambers simultaneously, while maintaining your breath at a steady tempo.

Please note that performance of the preceding perineal squeeze does, in fact, constitute a meditative act, which must not be practiced (again) if you want to avoid the blissful starkness of enlightenment.

Your perineum is also a key junction point in your meta-network of eight energy super conduits. You are already familiar with the approximately 2 inch diameter penetrating channel and how it runs from the perineum up and down the front face of your backbone, connecting the upper chamber in the center of your brain to the middle chamber in the center of your chest and the lower chamber in your lower abdomen; so let's now explore your super-conduit of maximum upward thrust.

Though energy will be discussed later in full, for now let's say that energy (chi) – the sensation of which, incidentally, you will have already experienced internally if you experimented with the aforementioned long, slow perineal squeeze – can (like electricity) be divided into negative and positive, or as the Taoists would say, yin and yang. Your yin energy moves downwards and inwards thus enabling you to feel settled on the spot, while your yang energy moves upwards and outwards enabling you to get out of bed in the morning (or evening) and get active.

The penetrating channel conducts both yin and yang energy (down and up), the horizontal belt channel, which you'll come to soon, also conducts both (horizontally), but the other six are exclusively yin or yang conduits – three yin, three yang.

Of these yang energy conduits, the most important and one you could least live without, is the conduit of maximum upward thrust. Approximately 1 inch in diameter, it begins at your perineum and runs up the rear face of your backbone all the way into your upper brainstem, over the top of your brain and comes to rest just above the roof of your mouth in the region of your pituitary gland. Running up the back of your spine as it does, it carries the yang energy responsible for holding your entire frame upright, not just physically but spiritually too, enabling you to reach out and explore in your life so you don't fester and become a potato. It is, in short, the super-conduit of maximum upward thrust. And if you wish to maintain (the illusion) of forward momentum as you hurtle round the sun, maintaining maximum upward thrust is a must. And to be able to trust that thrust, passage through the conduit must be unobstructed – passage, that is, for your awareness to travel freely up its length.

To that end, you may wish to pause momentarily to let awareness move backwards from your perineum into the conduit and upwards along the rear of your spinal column, over your brain, and into the pituitary region above the roof of your mouth. You can assist the ascent by squeezing the perineum as previously described, for the duration of the ascent and by remaining conscious of your breathing. You can either breathe in for the duration of the ascent and breathe out for the descent to be described imminently, or use the breath in the manner of a hydraulic pump, with each inhalation and exhalation jacking the awareness incrementally higher and higher up the conduit. It is quite normal to experience blockages along the route, which cause your mind to wander, but with gentle persistence the conduit will clear, facilitating a thrust you can trust. However, be sure to remain in the position of observing the entire procedure from your upper chamber, feeling it from the middle and driving it from the lower, otherwise you risk losing yourself in the motion.

But first, a short respite, a little breather to lighten things up a bit, here in the gap between the yang and the yin. Simply breathe slowly, imagining cosmic light in all the colors of the rainbow entering your body through every pore in your skin as you inhale, reaching your core (your three inner chambers), where the multi-hued light is purified and turned brilliant white. As you exhale, imagine this white light radiating outwards to the surface of your body and leaving through the pores of your skin to form a protective aura of white light extending up to 6 feet from your body all around, above and below you. Alternatively, situate yourself comfortably in your upper chamber and visualize a large, clear, uncut diamond of the highest quality suspended in inner space rotating slowly before your line of vision, lit from within by the same bright light you would have used to bolster your aura during the previous suggestion.

And now back to the main story line, which most recently had you poised suspended just above the roof of your mouth. What goes up must come down. This is true for energy as much as for apples or other solid objects. Starting just above the roof of your mouth, where the previous conduit stops, is the conduit of maximum downward drop, responsible for the main downward drop of yin energy.

It is this yin energy that is responsible for making you rest, sleep or remain still when necessary. Without it your yang energy, thrusting ever upwards as is its wont, will soon burn out.

If the yang energy thrusting upwards is responsible for holding everything up that requires upholding, such as your skeleton, internal organs, venous blood and flesh (hence why your flesh sags as you age and the yang naturally decreases), the yin energy dropping down is responsible for enabling everything that needs to drop to do so, such as digestive waste (elimination), pride, anger and other raging emotions, and even stupid ideas.

Achieving the balance between these two forces is every warrior's dream. It is effected by regular internal excursions along the lines currently being laid out in front of you.

To this effect, the super-conduit of maximum downward drop is also of approximately 1 inch diameter and runs down through the back of your throat, dropping like a plumb line behind your chest (in front of the penetrating channel), through your upper and lower abdomen, behind your pubic bone and ending in the perineum where the previous conduit begins, thus to form a loop. Just as when mentally tracing your way up the conduit of maximum upward thrust, be sure to maintain awareness in your three inner chambers simultaneously. If you used the perineal squeeze to help push your mind up the upward thrust regulator channel, release it now to allow the energy to drop back down the channel of maximum downward drop. Additionally, if you previously breathed in to lift the mind up in the ascent, breathe out now to facilitate its descent. Alternatively use the breath like a hydraulic pump as before, letting each inhalation and exhalation cycle push the awareness further and further down the conduit.

Rotating a portion of consciousness around this loop continually is a fundamental Taoist enlightenment trigger. Only practice it repeatedly if wishing to dramatically increase inner and outer strength and feelings of completeness and wellbeing. After completing at least one loop, rest for a moment to regroup at the perineum, breathing gently in and out and settle yourself within your three inner chambers, ready for the next phase of the journey.

SHORT INTERMISSION BEFORE MOVING DEEPER

While it is ideal from a warrior-quality-building point of view to stay focused on the inner process, you are after all human and therefore given to yearning for distraction. Rather than fight the urge, go with it. Unlike most other inner disciplines, Taoism insists you go with your human urges, indulge in the realm of the senses, let yourself wander like a child in the world of 10 thousand things. But as you do so, always maintain at least a minimum presence in your three inner chambers. Moreover, always remember to keep your breath flowing and your frame relaxed and at maximum expansion. This way even as you immerse yourself in distraction, you remain partly rooted in the undifferentiated absolute – the Tao.

In other words, as you saunter off now to make a cup of tea, watch TV, make a phone call, send an email or text message, ingest mind-altering substances or engage in mindless or meaningful sex (interact externally in other words), you will do so mindful and respectful of the underlying pattern which connects you to everyone and everything around you and will thus spiritualize your external experience. (N B: only apply this advice to all breaks taken from the inner process from now on if you want to perpetuate a constant state of enlightenment.)

So now, if sufficiently satiated on distraction, let us return to the plot without further ado.

MOVING INTO YOUR UPWARD THRUST REGULATOR CHANNEL, INCLUDING A BRIEF TRIP ROUND YOUR HORIZONTAL BELT CHANNEL

Your horizontal belt channel is the only energy meridian in the entire psychophysical system. It runs, as would a belt, around your waist, originating on your backbone from a point on the super-conduit of maximum upward thrust, level with your navel. It transports energy in both directions – clockwise and anticlockwise simultaneously.

It's job energetically is to hold you together (just like a belt) – and stop your trousers falling down – it stops you losing energy flow to the lower parts and legs in other words - it keeps it circulating.

When the energy is circulating fully here, the autonomic system has better control over all functions associated with the lower abdomen, pelvis, hips, legs and feet. This so on both the physical level – elimination, sexual drive, walking and so on, on the one hand, and the related psycho-emotional functions and conditions, feeling grounded (for the energy flowing to the feet), being able to let go of unhealthy prejudices, thoughts and beliefs (elimination), having the strength of mind to step boldly into new situations – and back out again if the situation's not feeling right to you (energy moving through the legs).

Activate the belt channel now by (visualizing) breathing in through the spine between the vertebrae at waist height, gathering the breath at that point for a moment and as you exhale, sending the breath in two streams, one left, one right, round to the front, like a belt made of light, meeting just below the navel like a bright shiny buckle, getting brighter with each breath.

Do nine breaths' worth of this, then reverse it: breathe in through that point just below the navel then breathe it out from there round to the back again – again nine times.

This simultaneous flow of yin and yang energy around the horizontal is responsible for joining the energy of the upper body with the energy of the lower, for stimulating and protecting the fire in your lower chamber and for overseeing events in the reproductive organs. Only revolve your mind round this channel continuously, in both directions simultaneously, if wishing to develop an unassailable protective energy sheath or if wishing to restore the generative fire in the lower chamber after a hard night (or day) of sex or after a particularly expensive shopping expedition. Climbing slowly up the super-conduit of maximum downward drop is a little like walking up the down escalators – it's fun and it makes your legs stronger, but requires extra attention lest you get swept down before reaching where you want to go. In this case, that is a point 2 inches below the navel about 1 inch under the surface, where the maximum downward drop conduit is traversed by the horizontal belt channel.

At this intersection, your awareness divides in two to travel round the belt channel in both directions simultaneously. They nearly meet again where the belt channel traverses the super conduit of maximum upward thrust, on the rear face of your backbone at the level of the navel. Except they don't. Instead, you stop 2 inches either side of that intersection in order to join the upward thrust regulator channel. This channel is approximately 1 inch diameter and originates bilaterally in the balls of your feet. It travels bilaterally up the inside of your legs, becomes one stream at the perineum, where it divides again moving bilaterally up your back outwards in a roughly diagonal direction like a pair of braces to the tip of each shoulder, intersecting the horizontal belt channel at waist level.

So there you were waiting patiently on the horizontal belt channel 2 inches either side of the spine where the upward regulator channel intersects the belt channel. Continue now bilaterally up each of the two strands till you reach your shoulder tips, where the channel runs bilaterally down the center of the outside of each arm, to the end of each index finger and back into the center of each palm. As before, make use of the previously described perineal squeeze and breathing options to augment your momentum. Rest now for a moment in the center of each palm, maintaining a simultaneous minimum presence in your three inner chambers and breathing freely. It's time to join your downward drop energy regulator channel. (Any directional discrepancy you may be about to perceive will be quickly remedied by visualizing your arms held vertically up above your head. You'll see what I mean.)

JOINING YOUR DOWNWARD DROP ENERGY REGULATOR CHANNEL

Starting in the center of each palm (points, by the way, that when energetically activated render you more generous, loving and able to transmit healing energy through your palms for others' benefit) allow your mind to travel bilaterally up the midline of the soft underside of each arm and into the deepest point in each armpit (points that when activated stimulate your middle chamber thus increasing your ability to feel). From here, the channel drops bilaterally down the front of your torso in an inwardly diagonal direction like the front section of your trouser braces to intersect your horizontal belt channel at waist level.

The channel itself continues all the way to the perineum, separates over the top of the thighs and travels down the outside of each leg to the end of the second toes and back into the ball of each foot to join the start of the upward thrust regulator channel. For now, however, your awareness leaves the channel at the intersection with your belt channel at waist level, two inches either side of the Midline, whence it circulates simultaneously in both directions on the horizontal to meet on the spine at the intersection with the super-conduit of maximum upward thrust at navel height.

Now comes another moment of moving against the flow, this time walking down an up elevator, as your awareness drops down the super-conduit of maximum upward thrust into the perineum, where you stop and make another cup of tea or equivalent before re-entering your penetrating channel.

RE-ENTERING YOUR PENETRATING CHANNEL, SUBSEQUENTLY TO PLUNGE YOURSELF SWIFTLY DOWNWARDS

From your perineum, you're going to gain a little altitude now to facilitate a proper drop down to your feet. Before you do, take a moment to reassemble yourself in your three inner chambers – observing the proceedings from the upper chamber, feeling them warmly from the middle and driving the entire experience from the lower, all the while breathing freely, slowly and deeply, with physical frame at comfortable maximum expansion and all muscles completely relaxed. If distracting thoughts persist, spend a moment focused in your upper chamber translating those thoughts into visual shapes appearing from nowhere, dancing across the screen on the back of the forehead in front of you and disappearing again into nowhere. If this doesn't work and you still find your mind all jumbled, visualize that clear, uncut, internally lit diamond rotating slowly in your upper chamber.

This, by the way, is one of the fastest and most effective methods known to humankind for clearing the mind of unwanted mental distraction, other than a full lobotomy or decapitation.

Having thus regrouped, using the perineal squeeze and breathe options as before if you want, let awareness slowly ascend your penetrating channel from your perineum up to the level of your solar plexus (major nerve plexus in your upper abdomen). Be sure to stop below chest level, as the energy generated by your momentum (up to now touring your internal architecture) could overload your middle chamber at this point and become trapped there, possibly causing heart problems.

Your solar plexus, incidentally, is associated as its name implies with the sun, bright light, happiness and success. It is said (by me and other preceding Taoists) that visualizing the midday sun shining brilliantly in your solar plexus at all times will ensure your constant cheerfulness, positivity and success in worldly matters. You should not practice this visualization if wishing to remain miserable, wretched or unsuccessful – it's not a visualization for losers, in other words.

From your solar plexus, or 'yellow palace' as those Taoist romantics of old were sometimes known to call it (probably after one too many psychoactive mushrooms), you are about to let yourself plunge as if by bungee down through your penetrating channel to your perineum. Here, fast downward momentum forces awareness to divide in two and dart bilaterally outwards along your inguinal canals (those grooves running from your pubic bone across the tops of your thighs where they join with your lower abdomen), to your outer hip joints. From your outer hip joints, awareness plunges bilaterally down the outside of your legs through your downward drop regulator channel past your outer ankle joints, over the dorsum of your feet to the end of your second toes and back into the ball of each foot to join the start of your upward thrust regulator channel.

Downwardly plunging yourself thus, while remaining assembled in your three inner chambers, assisted by full exhalation and total muscular release of the pelvic floor, is incidentally a most sound method of grounding or rooting yourself in a hurry, to be used whenever your emotions are in turmoil or your mind is spinning out of control in the midst of a busy day (or night).

ASCENT THROUGH YOUR UPWARD THRUST REGULATOR CHANNEL

What goes down, must come up. Remembering yourself yet again in your three inner chambers, and taking advantage of the perineal squeeze and breathing options (breathing in for the duration of the ascent or breathing in and out to generate the sensation of a hydraulic pump), let your awareness rise up through your upward thrust regulator channel, which starts in the balls of your feet, runs back bilaterally under your inner ankle joints, up the inside of your legs and into your perineum. At this juncture you leave your upward thrust regulator channel and walk the wrong way up the down escalator through your super-conduit of maximum downward drop, up to the aforementioned point 2 inches below your navel.

This point represents the front door of the lower chamber and is the point focused on as an instant centring device by practitioners of the strongly recommended Taoist martial arts (tai-chi, hsing-i and pa-kua), and is coincidentally associated with material wealth. Only spend time focusing on it while visualizing money attracted to it at high velocity (and in high denomination notes), from all directions simultaneously, if wishing to instantaneously manifest large sums of money in your life or if wishing to center yourself while engaged in self-defense or other extreme sports.

From here, drop your awareness back down to your perineum and reassemble yourself in your three inner chambers, checking your breathing for fluidity, tempo and depth and your mainframe for optimum vertical and horizontal expansion. (Rest assured, by the way, that my constant repetition of basic instructions is intended to institute an automatic pattern of return to your core – the inner chambers – with regular frequency from now on and does not in any way imply that I think you may be thick.)

RETURNING TO VERTICAL LOOP MODE

Let your awareness return once again now to your super-conduit of maximum upward thrust, travelling up the rear face of your backbone, over the top of your brain, behind your forehead to rest just above the roof of your mouth. You can assist the ascent by squeezing your perineum and breathing in for the duration of the ascent, or by using a succession of in and out breaths as a hydraulic pump.

From the area above the roof of your mouth, let awareness drop down behind your throat, chest, through your belly, behind your pubic bone and back into your perineum. You can assist the descent by releasing your perineum and exhaling for the duration of the drop, or by using the breath as a hydraulic pump as before.

It is never good for purposes of on-the-spot yin-yang harmonization to return to this basic vertical loop as often as possible both during such sessions of internal exploration and whilst in interaction with your external world during the course of a busy schedule, unless you truly want to feel powerful.

But there's a way to go yet before completing the tour (whereupon its true purpose and value will be revealed).

ANOTHER DOWNWARD PLUNGE

From your perineum, let your awareness climb up the down escalator in your super-conduit of maximum downward drop to the aforementioned point 2 inches below your navel to instigate a catapult effect. This subsequently sends your awareness down through your perineum, thence to divide into two streams running bilaterally outwards along the grooves of the inguinal canals (that connect your upper thighs to your torso), to the outer hip bones to join your downward thrust regulator channel and continue bilaterally down the outside of your legs, under your outer ankle joints, to the end of your second toes, finally coming to rest in the balls of your feet. Repeal your self-assemblage process in your three inner chambers, check your breathing, expand and relax.

AND THRUST UP AGAIN

From the balls of your feet, let awareness travel back along your upward thrust regulator channel, under your inner ankle joints, rising up the inside of your legs to your perineum.

The next bit is kind of intimate, so check no one's looking over your shoulder as you read this.

There are a pair of secondary channels, extensions in fact of your super-conduits of maximum upward thrust and maximum downward drop. One starts in your perineum, and runs just beneath the skin's surface up to the tip of your uterus (if you're currently female). From your uterus a downwardly plunging channel runs back (down) to your perineum. (If currently male), the one mirroring your upward thrust regulator channel begins at your perineum, runs just beneath the skin's surface along the length of the front of your penis (when looking in the mirror at your penis in flaccid mode), to the penile tip. From the tip of your penis, a second channel runs up the underside of your penis (when in flaccid mode) back to your perineum.

Activating these channels was a device used in secret Taoist societies concerned with producing enlightenment through sex. It was soon discovered that such self-activation would produce interesting results, not least of which were a noticeable increase in sexual vigor (responsible for staying power and orgasm amplification) as well as sexual magnetism (pulling power, in other words).

You should therefore not attempt self-activation of these genital channels if wishing to preserve yourself in a state of celibacy or chasteness, or if wishing not to meet new potential lovers. Otherwise, let awareness travel slowly from your perineum to the tip of your uterus or penis (depending on how you currently stand gender-wise) on the exhalation and from the tip of said uterus or penis back to your perineum. Remember that countless repetitions of the above will eventually get you in trouble.

To add to potential trouble, make use of the perineal squeeze option, squeezing as awareness travels to the uterine or penile tip and releasing as it returns perineum-wards.

The purpose of activating these channels here, however, is not primarily to spice up your love life, but to stimulate and gather your primal essence (traditionally known as jing) in order that it may be refined in the next phase of the internal process into higher-grade energy (chi). This chi will then be refined further into spirit, but spirit in a localized, microcosmic sense (equating to soul in Western cosmology). Microcosmic spirit, or soul, will then be transmuted into macrocosmic spirit, as in Great Spirit – or Tao, in other words. When this happens, you momentarily transcend all sense of local self (or selves) in one blissful instant, which is not only a fulfilling and existentially reassuring experience while in deep contemplation but can also be employed as a workaday tool in normal street life to effect an external change of conditions.

The following should therefore be ignored if you would rather not hold the keys to indulging in the Taoist tradition of 'wu wei', the art of manifesting what you need in the physical world without strain of effort – as if by magic, in other words.

RETURN TO YOUR PENETRATING CHANNEL

Having made the genital excursion and returned safely to your perineum, ensuring as always that a modicum of presence is being maintained within your three inner chambers, that your mainframe is at maximum expansion and that your breath is fluid, even and deep, re-enter your penetrating channel. Let awareness travel up to the rear door of your lower chamber (level with your navel on the front of your spine). Enter through the rear door and, looking in for a moment, spread yourself once around the 'walls'. Float back through the door and continue upwards till you arrive at the back door of your middle chamber (at center-chest level on the front face of your backbone), entering, spreading and floating out again likewise. From here keep climbing until you reach the back door of the upper chamber, repeating entering and spreading procedures, but delaying egress for some moments, while we regroup and take stock.

It is an empirical rule in Taoist philosophy that where your thoughts go, your energy (chi) follows.

What has just occurred, therefore, almost without you realizing, is that you have gathered your intensified primal essence through the previous genital channel excursion, drawn it up into your inner chamber where it was transmuted into more refined energy (known traditionally as the 'pill of immortality'), drawn that 'pill' up into your middle chamber where it was transmuted into microcosmic spirit or 'soul', and finally drawn that soul up to your upper chamber, where it has now been transmuted into pure spirit, or Tao.

Or at least it would be it I wasn't going on in your ear and distracting you like this. You might perhaps like to take a closed eye moment on your own to contemplate this before continuing. While you do, be sure to enhance the experience by visualizing the crown of your head open to the sky and, by extension, the cosmos above and around you.

While thus contemplating, allow yourself the momentary sense of being connected to the entirety of existence, that union being unobstructed by any previously imagined barriers or limitations.

The sublimity of this internal experience is as ineffable as the Tao itself and would satiate all but the most seasoned psychonaut. It would suffice for you too, were it not for your urban warrior aspirations, which dictate that you must be able to transport this entire experience into the external realm of moment-to-moment life out on the high street. For this very purpose the Tao thoughtfully provided you with what is traditionally known to Taoists as a 'spirit body'.

SPIRIT BODY!

Aye, a spirit body.

And what it is, is an etheric shape or mainframe existing in the same space as your physical body (though rather more expansive), designed to maintain the integrity of your consciousness as an ongoing entity from the point of physical death onwards. It is also used to protect your consciousness, or spirit, and by extension your physical body while still alive – especially when in physical danger, indulging in astral travel or engaged in the practice of wu wei or changing of external conditions through 'magic'.

All preceding self-exploration of your internal somatic architecture has in fact been in order to define and realize the anatomy of your spirit body, which you would do well to acknowledge now (before offence is taken – spirits can be temperamental too), by letting your awareness plunge back down to your perineum with a hearty exhalation. At the point of impact between plunging awareness and perineum, allow yourself an instant of spirit body recognition, experiencing yourself as possessed of limitless power, absolute harmony and eternal duration, those qualities subtly encased within a unified and integrated etheric form.

Allow this form (your spirit body, in case you were getting lost in weighty abstractions just then), to expand and grow so large it encompasses the entire known universe and everything in it. While involved in social intercourse with polite company, however, allow yourself to expand only enough to fill the room or space in which your interaction is taking place.

While consciously identifying with your spirit body, imbibe the quality of limitless power into your lower chamber, absolute harmony into your middle chamber and eternal duration into your upper chamber. Remember, your spirit body is not an identity to foster unless you want to be able to effect radical transformation of external conditions at will and without effort, or unless you want to be well-prepared for death (in other words, only consciously foster this identity if wishing to experience moment-lo-moment existence from the perspective of an immortal spirit).

Sit for a while now contemplating these abstractions: the vastness of limitless power contained within your belly, the perfection of absolute harmony contained within your chest and the magnitude of eternal duration contained within the center of your brain.

As you sit containing these qualities within your inner chambers, allow yourself the existential luxury of the sensation of limitlessness, so that you become, or at least feel, unified with the limitless Tao itself – these qualities being coincidentally fundamental to the Tao as well as your own personal immortal spirit.

Now, if in this state of identification with your spirit body you wish to be able to alter external conditions without effort (in other words, manifest something you need on the material plane), simply allow awareness to travel from your perineum up your super-conduit of maximum upward thrust (along the rear face of your spine) to that point in the center of the base of your skull where flesh meets bone. It is through this point (the rear door of your cavity of original consciousness) that cosmic energy enters your spirit body. Spend a moment feeling the influx, then let your now cosmically charged awareness travel forward (through the super-conduit of maximum upward thrust) over the top of your brain and down into the center of your forehead, just above the bridge of your nose.

With awareness thus held, simultaneously reassemble yourself within your three inner chambers and project onto the screen on the back of the forehead in front of you a clear image or symbol of what it is you require to be made manifest in real time.

This is not the time or place to go into the morals and ethics appertaining to manifestation through magic, save to say that, according to the universal and immutable law of cause and effect, if you attempt by magic to entrap or adversely influence or coerce another human being in any scenario not by their free will or for their highest possible good, you will soon find yourself similarly entrapped, adversely influenced or coerced, because that's the way magic works. So, to save time (because, in case we forget, there isn't any), let me simply say, for your own sake, don't.

Conversely, healing wishes sent to another individual or grouping of individuals from this spiritually identified space will also rebound on your person, but this time with beneficial results commensurate with the intensity of the original outward-bound thought.

There are enough self-help books around to help you to assimilate the ethics and practice of visualization without us having to waste further time on the subject at this point.

But whichever way you decide to call it, hold the image of what you want to be made manifest dearly in focus on the screen in front of you. Consciously dispel the essence of any self-limiting factors such as guilt, unworthiness, anxiety, doubt, self-recrimination and any other self-restricting superstition you have been unconsciously harboring that could possibly hinder or block altogether the manifestation process. For dispelling purposes, it helps to internally gather up all negative qualifies as you breathe in and to see yourself releasing them as you breathe out. You may find it necessary to complete up to nine full breath cycles before feeling satisfied that all self-limiting energy has been expunged.

WELCOMING IN THE SPIRITS

As a spirit yourself in this state of identifying fully with your spirit body in other words – you are perfectly at liberty to call in other spirits for a cup of spiritual tea of an afternoon.

Welcome in the spirit of abundance. Welcome in the spirit of compatible companionship. Welcome in the spirit of health and longevity. Welcome in the spirit of love. Welcome in the spirit of enlightenment. Welcome in the spirit of success. Welcome in the spirit of fun. And above ail welcome in the spirit of humor, without which we'd have no comedians, no politicians (though of course these are often interchangeable) and no barefoot doctors spilling the beans so freely.

Bask in the internal glow brought about by the arrival into your orbit of such spirits as you deem fit to invite, and fully imbibe the essence of the gift each one brings you. The more fully you imbibe, the more substantial will be the material manifestations of those gifts (in real time).

MOMENTARY CLOSURE

To complete the metaphysical loop now, with desired essences gathered within, let your awareness plunge down your super-conduit of maximum downward drop, from the middle of your forehead, just above the bridge of your nose, where it has been waiting politely for me to continue, all the way down through the back of your throat, behind your chest, through your upper and lower abdomen, behind your pubic bone and into your perineum, which is probably getting quite worn out by now, so let's stop and give it a rest, while we make a brief detour into a fuller explanation of energy and the essential role it plays in all this spiritual malarkey.

YOUR ENERGY AND YOU

Well here you are, about as deep as a person can go existentially without actually being swallowed up by the ground. At this point it would be inappropriate of me not to elucidate further upon the slippery business of energy and to hopefully allude to its nature successfully enough to inspire you to understand more about it and to help you experience more of it on a moment- to-moment basis.

As I've already stated, the first empirical rule is that where your thought goes your energy will follow. If, for example, you think of your right hand, energy will instantaneously flow into that hand. Think of your left foot and energy will flow into it. Think of someone you love and energy, which after all is not restricted by physical bounds, will flow (on a subtle level) towards them. This is what gives thoughts their power to make things manifest (by wu wei), which is why it always pays to be clear about what thoughts you're breathing life into.

I mention breathing here because the second empirical rule states by linking mind and breath, your power of thought is exponentially multiplied.

Test this on your right hand now. Quickly center yourself, assembling your awareness within your three inner chambers and hold your breath (for a brief moment) while concentrating on your hand, noting whatever sensation arises there. Now breathe out, imagining the breath flowing down the outside of your right arm to the end of your second finger and back into the center of your palm, noting the sensation. You may notice sensation is stronger and awareness more defined when you breathe (life) into your palm than when your breath is held. (This technique, incidentally, of breathing into the palm, is employed by practitioners of Taoist healing during the laying on oi hands, as well as by practitioners of the [yet again] highly recommended Taoist martial arts [tai-chi, pa-kua and hsing-i], both offensively to project and deliver amplified 'striking' energy through the palm, fist, or any other striking surface - including feet, knees, elbows, shoulders, foreheads and weapons – and defensively to amplify protection of any particular body part or parts when being struck.)

The same applies when sending a thought (and therefore energy) to someone through the ether for purposes of say healing or establishing telepathic contact for any other reason (such as sudden unexpected mobile phone battery death while out and about). If when sending the thought, you breathe out, imagining the breath transporting your thought to its desired destination, you will magnify that thought's definition, power and effect.

The third empirical rule states that when your thought or thoughts are cheerful, your energy will be light and will vibrate at high frequency, thus finding resonance (by the immutable law of affinity) with others whose vibrational rate matches your own. In practice, this means that wherever you go others will be kindly disposed towards you and your mutual cheerfulness will produce synergy, which will obviously help things run more smoothly for you whether at work, rest or play.

By the same token, when your thoughts are glum, your energy will be turgid, heavy and of low vibrational frequency, so finding resonance (by the same immutable law of affinity) with others of similar vibrational rate. In practice, this means encountering miserable bastards wherever you go, whose glumness mixed with yours will produce entropy, thus causing obstruction to your easy passage through the course of a day. This is why it's important, if you like things smooth and easy, to remind yourself to remain cheerful at all times no matter what. And if you need a prop, just think of your good fortune for not having been flattened by an Earthbound passing asteroid, swallowed by a suddenly re-emerging galactic black hole or swept 80 miles out to sea by a surprise tidal wave yet today – immediately desist from self- pity and appreciate your blessings, in other words.

When you have suffered illness, a protracted phase of unhealthy living (hammering it, in other words), receipt of bad news or any other overwhelming accumulation of external pressure upon your person, your energy becomes strained and decreases in vibrational frequency, thus making your thoughts gloomy in general and hence instigating a negative spiral.

Fortunately, when your energy is light and vibrating at high frequency, as a result of exercise, a phase of healthy living or in fact engaging in any uplifting activity, reading this book at this very moment for example, your thoughts will be cheerful, thus instigating a positive spiral.

But initially, at least as far as you're concerned here and now on the planet, all past-life karma and untoward environmental considerations taken into account, every process begins with a thought.

Which is why (I repeat) it's crucial if you want a positive outcome, to be of cheerful intent at every point in the process (of life).

So energy follows thought. OK. But what actually is it?

For a full and proper explanation, firstly consult Einstein or any available nearby competent physicist, who would no doubt be able to enlighten you on the subject far more eloquently and succinctly than this scientifically untutored barefoot doctor.

However, if such consultation should prove difficult to arrange or insert into your already full agenda, hopefully the following will temporarily suffice.

Energy is the life-blood of the universe

In fact, it is the very foundation of all existence itself. If the Tao is the context in which all of life is framed, energy is the active agent that effects the arisal and dispersal of all phenomena. Energy is, in other words, the active agent of change and transformation both microcosmically and macrocosmically throughout existence (and non-existence).

Energy is not confined to the three-dimensional world, but coexists simultaneously in the fourth (time), fifth (spirit) and all dimensions beyond (currently ineffable). It doesn't need a time machine to traverse the aeons or a stick of incense to make itself feel spiritual.

Energy is ubiquitous and unbounded, though it will naturally channel itself through specific pathways wherever they present themselves in objects or phenomena with which it interacts.

Energy is innately intelligent. It carries encoded seminal data, which it imparts as a template for transformation to everything through or upon which it acts.

Energy rising up through the frequency spectrum is positive, creative or yang and the transformational template it imparts promotes positive growth in all it interacts with.

Energy moving down through the frequency spectrum is negative, destructive or yin and produces entropy in all it interacts with.

It should be noted that yin and yang are terms relative to each other and the context in which they're used and should not be mistaken for definitions of creative and destructive functions, except in the extreme. Yin represents the passive state where yang represents the active. Passivity in its extreme static state leads to stagnation, which leads in turn to dissolution. Activity in its extreme hypermotile state leads to combustion and therefore also to dissolution.

Normally, except in the extreme (moments of birth or death – of anything including slugs, people, planets, solar systems or so on), energy is moving both ways through the spectrum more or less evenly, which providing the balance is tilted at least 51 per cent towards the positive (upward, yang thrust) will act as a catalyst for healthy growth in whichever medium it flows through. As soon as this balance tilts the other way, however, its action becomes anabolic instead.

Energy vibrates at varying frequency. The slower the rate of vibration, the more it transforms into solid matter. At the negative end of the spectrum, in its most inert state, energy takes shape as anti-matter (black holes or the Taoist concept of non-existence). As its frequency of vibrational rate increases in the spectrum, it manifests in mineral form as rock and other such coalescences of (apparently) inert matter, progressing from primordial slime all the way up the evolutionary scale to mammalian state. As it continues to rise beyond this through the spectrum, it becomes increasingly more pure and refined in manifestation (electricity, sound, light, ether, thought, spirit and beyond) as its vibrational rate accelerates. Thought, therefore, travels faster than an email (currently 3,000 miles per second) and even faster than the speed of light (186,000 miles per second). Theoretically this means someone having afternoon tea on a planet in the vicinity of Sirius can receive a thought from you almost instantaneously, eight and a half years before they could see you waving. That's how fast energy moves when manifesting as thought. Obviously the same theoretical result cannot be guaranteed if that person is drinking absinthe – something a person may well develop a weakness for if spatially marooned in such far-flung locales.

Although universally ubiquitous and all-powerful, energy can be induced (and indeed very much enjoys being so induced), to channel itself along specific pathways within and around your own body in response to commands from your mind.

When energy flowing through your body is positively activated by your mind, which incidentally is what you were doing while taking the preceding grand tour of your own internal somatic architecture, it acquires the strength of refined steel, as the Taoist martial artists would put it. And it is this refined strength that lends itself to providing all the 'superhuman', 'supernatural' powers (self-regeneration, self-defense, self-actualization, instantaneous wish- realization, overwhelming charisma, healing powers, spiritual enlightenment and so on) that every urban warrior loves so much.

Psychoactively charged energy is commonly referred to as 'chi' or 'qi' – though the word has no sacred or magical significance in itself (unless you're in the business of bottling it and need to trademark a name).

But in case we forget, under the amnesia-inducing effect of the combined weight of the foregoing collection of hefty abstractions, chi is a physical phenomenon capable of imparting not only the universal transformational template, but immense bliss on a personal moment- to-moment basis too.

To demonstrate, let me invite the small child in you to partake in the momentary pleasures of developing a one-to-one relationship with the following 'toy'.

YOUR INVISIBLE MORPHING GOLDEN BALL

Where your mind goes, your energy follows. In light of how energy transforms itself into varying degrees of matter depending on its vibrational frequency, this implies that you can create whatever you want with your thoughts.

This is tantamount to saying you create your own reality or that you create reality with your belief, but let's leave such grandiose claims to one side for now and stick to specifics.

Obviously there will be a delay in real-time manifestation while thought and energy project themselves into the ether to undergo the necessary electrochemical process and pick up the requisite offal dust or whatever they use over there to solidify enough to drop back down to Earth some time later as substantial events in real time.

The length of this delay depends on a host of variables, not least of which are the clarity of your initial intent, the actual viability of what you're wishing for, the degree of concurrence of your wishes with the natural flow or Tao in the greater scheme of things, the volume of outbound wish-traffic to be processed, and the levels of resistance you may be harboring unconsciously to actually materializing what you want. Arising from low self-esteem, feelings of unworthiness or superstitious belief in a god that wants you to suffer, this unconscious resistance will corrupt the purity, clarity and definition of the outward bound wish, with ensuing confusion on the etheric plane while 'they' work out whether you want what you wish for or not. I say 'they', but of course it's actually you, or that part of you that exists in the ether – Big You, in other words.

In this instant, however, what you are about to create is pretty close to hand, fairly modest in scope and should therefore materialize before your very eyes, albeit invisibly, with very little delay indeed.

Assemble yourself in triplicate within your three inner chambers, checking briefly for maximum mainframe expansion (sit up straight in other words), relaxation and sinking of the flesh, and depth, evenness and fluidity of breath. Pay extra attention to broadening and relaxing across your upper back and shoulders, as well as softening your arms.

Raise your hands, palms touching, in 'prayer* position to the level of your solar plexus (upper abdomen). Keep your elbows away from your sides to make space in your armpits, referred to by Taoists of poetic bent as 'holding golden apples' (in your armpits).

Maintaining a minimum diplomatic presence in your inner chambers, send a thought to your palms commanding them to feel magnetically connected to each other. Slowly and sensitively separate your palms 3 inches. Now just as slowly close the gap down to 1 inch. Repeat this action nine times or so, concentrating on the magnetism between your hands.

Once this sensation of magnetism is satisfactorily established, open your palms to a distance of approximately 8 inches. Imagine you're holding an invisible golden ball capable of expanding or contracting to fit between your palms, no matter how close or far apart, regardless of the position you're holding them relative to the rest of your body.

Now with your palms 8 inches apart, slowly and sensitively raise them to chest level then lower them to navel level concentrating all the while on the magnetic connection you are creating between them – the invisible morphing golden ball, in other words.

Repeat this nine times in the manner of a male giant languidly masturbating (of an afternoon), paying attention now not only to the magnetism contained in the ball, but also to (the sensation of) magnetic resonance in your lower and middle chambers as the giant slowly bashes away metaphorically at his bishop. Note the energetic sensations in your belly and chest, in other words as the ball moves up and down.

Now (checking once again for maximum mainframe expansion, relaxation, sinking, breathing and inner chamber occupancy levels) lower both palms to navel level, turned slightly skywards and approximately 6 inches apart as if cupping the ball from below. Slowly (and sensitively) move the ball through an anticlockwise circle on the horizontal plane in front of you in the manner of the Earth's heliocentric orbit (orbiting the sun) minus its axial rotation and tilt.

Complete nine anticlockwise orbits and nine clockwise orbits concentrating on both the ball and its magnetic pull in your lower chamber. Now repeat this in both directions at chest height with palms turned down towards the floor, as if the ball is underneath sticking to your palms.

Now lower the ball to navel height and push it slowly diagonally upwards away from you in the manner of a small child handing a ball to someone taller. When your arms are nearly at full extension, draw the ball back towards your chest and slide it down the front of your body to navel height, thus to form a circular trajectory, along which you then proceed to turn the ball, rather in the manner of a soldier before a big parade wiping round the circumference of the bass drum strapped to his front with both palms simultaneously. After nine revolutions change direction and repeat.

Now hold the ball at navel height with right hand uppermost and left hand lowermost. Slowly rotate the ball, allowing your forearms to swivel fluidly until your left hand is uppermost. And then the other way and so on until you complete approximately nine cycles, remaining mindful of the sensations of magnetic resonance in your lower and middle chambers.

Now hold the ball above the crown of your head as if about to throw it into the distance. Instead of which, you open the gap between your palms to allow the ball to expand to a diameter of approximately 18 inches, then close the gap to compress the ball to a diameter of only 1 inch, all the while remaining mindful of the sensations of magnetic resonance in your upper chamber. By now you will have had enough time to establish the foundations for a comfortable relationship with your invisible morphing golden ball, at least sufficient to encourage you to experiment with some improvised moves of your own.

For as you've probably worked out, it's not the moves that count, but the generation of magnetically resonant field (energy or chi, in other words), both between your palms and simultaneously within your three inner chambers.

Simply by waving it around a bit in the air, this way or that, your invisible morphing golden ball becomes a (literally) handy energy battery at your disposal. The energy generated with all this ball action not only provides sensual pleasure, but also provides a tangible experience of the intangible – no mean feat!

My purpose for introducing it at this stage of the proceedings is twofold. Firstly, it provides a welcome interlude of non-heady, body-centered experience, which is always a healing thing to do. And secondly and more importantly, it provides an experiential reference point with regard to your energy and what it feels like, which will be useful in the next stages of internal exploration.

Meantime, it's perfectly OK to practice your ball maneuvers in public – just keep the ball small and your movements discreet, as if gently exercising your wrists, and no one will think anything of it – at the most they may think you've got a mild slow-motion twitch, but what do you care!

BEING CLEAR WITH YOURSELF - SYNERGY AND YOU

Energy is consciousness in motion. It follows your intention. Every known phenomenon is subject to change. All phenomena arise as if from nowhere, each according to its own intrinsic blueprint or nature, and proceed to coagulate into various shapes. Sooner or later that shape disintegrates and the phenomenon eventually disappears into the void again – the seed of its destruction having been planted at its inception.

Energy is the active transformative agent acting through the phenomenon, the catalyst for that perpetual cycle contained within each phenomenon's intrinsic blueprint comprising birth, growth, maturity, decline and death. This implies receptivity and passivity of the phenomenon through which that energy is flowing.

However, when the receptive phenomenon in question happens to be you (you that is, who has (already) experienced what it is to actually hold that energy as per the preceding invisible golden morphing ball control practice, who has been familiarized with your internal somatic architecture within which that energy can be refined and amplified, and who has also instigated a connection with that stratum of (your) being that contemporaneously exists in the fifth dimension, where your consciousness is one and the same as the consciousness contained in energy – your spirit body in other words) then it is entirely possible (and advisable) for you to adopt a proactive role in relation to energy and how it acts upon your person.

In other words, what, as a warrior, you are internally training yourself to do (by this simple action of reading and assimilating) is to actually harness the transformative agent, energy – the primary cosmic force and the very lifeblood of the universe itself – and use it to effect changes in both internal and external conditions, according to your will.

When energy impacts on any phenomenon it causes transformation. If that phenomenon is fairly inert like a rock, there will be only minimum synergy produced by their meeting and the transformation will be slow (which is why it requires hundreds of millions of years for rocks to change shape, which is fine because most rocks are fairly patient by nature – not all though, so be on guard whenever trekking near major fault lines, actively volcanic terrain or high-mountain country after heavy rains).

However, when you, as identified with your spirit body, are the phenomenon through which energy flows, great synergy is produced on impact, leading to a rapid change of conditions.

Synergy, the phenomenon of, say, one hundred units of energy meeting another hundred units of energy and producing not two hundred, but a full one thousand units in total, multiplies itself by a series of quantum leaps.

Synergy is a way of describing the etheric field of infinite possibilities – a field of greater harmonic resonance in which your ideas or pictures, i.e. your wishes, are transformed in the fifth dimension into events, which then occur locally in dimensions one to four to be experienced by you on a sensual level in full detail.

Implied in the process of touring your internal somatic architecture is the subtle initiation of self as universal energy conductor.

As you increase your capacity to channel and amplify energy (as you continue reading) that energy will multiply itself and produce synergy. Synergy increases exponentially in direct proportion to the clarity of your intent.

So it is synergy that makes your dreams come true. The question is, what are your dreams?

BEING CLEAR WITH WHAT YOU WANT

During the course of the second tour of your internal architecture, which starts in but a few minutes depending on reading speed and availability (yours), you will activate the requisite synergy to make your dreams come true. (Though perhaps not in quite the way you think.)

This places a hefty responsibility on your metaphysical shoulders and requires that you follow certain principles if you want to avoid inadvertently manifesting what turns out to be a lousy or inappropriate dream.

Life here on the planet, as any butterfly who thinks he's a person dreaming he's a butterfly will tell you, is but a dream. Making your dreams come true implies, in a sense, changing one dream scenario for another (hopefully improved one). In so doing, the new scenario may well turn out subtly or even grossly different from how you imagined it would. Just like any dream, definition can be nebulous. But according to the empirical laws of wu wei (the aforementioned Taoist habit of materializing dreams without straining yourself), the essence you were yearning for will nonetheless materialize in the most appropriate form for you at exactly the time you need it. (That's how the Tao works if you're willing to trust it enough.)

Say, for example, you are dreaming of owning a grand house on a hill. What essence will owning that house bring you? A sense of security, satisfaction and peace, let's say. These then comprise the essence of the scenario you wish to materialize. The house on the hill you actually get through the wu wei habit may be physically quite different from the one in your fantasy, perhaps not as grand, perhaps grander, maybe on a different hill in a different country in a different phase of life altogether. But you will feel secure, accomplished and peaceful as you gaze out over the view from your veranda nevertheless. On the other hand, you may well get the exact house at precisely the time you want.

Anyway, the details are not important.

The essence is your call, the details work themselves out each according to its own innate Tao or blueprint of arisal and dispersal.

So what you do is use your mind to command 'your' energy to produce the desired somatic experience of the particular essence you want to introduce. If you want to introduce the essence of security, accomplishment and peace you think would come with owning that house on the hill for example, you simply invite that essence into your internal energy field by conscious command.

Once this essence is flowing within your internal meta-network (of eight super-conduits) it will find resonance through synergy in the ether where dreams actualize before taking shape in real time on the ground. And hey presto, synergy will manifest the one house on the one hill on the entire planet that could possibly fit the bill, providing exactly the right conditions for you to experience those essences in full detail and surround sound. It might even turn out to be the one house on the one hill on all the planet that doesn't get washed away under the sea.

But it won't matter to you that much either way, other than to confirm the efficacy of your wu wei practice, because you already contain the desired essence within. Not that you wouldn't appreciate it of course. As a warrior, you'd just be too damned centered in the moment to take that much notice of external conditions. Paradoxically, this very centeredness is what attracts the most advantageous external conditions anyway, so you're on to a winner whichever house you end up with. (The main thing is to have a roof over your head and at least one wall to hang your diplomas on.)

Urban warriors following the Tao do not play an end-game. End-games are pure Hollywoodism.

Hollywoodism is based on the illusory linear (straight line) model of measuring your life ahead of time by the projected achievement of a succession of external goals culminating in a happy ending, where death intrudes as a big shock and surprise.

Taoists, like physicists, say there are no straight lines in the universe, only curves. Extend any line far enough and it curves round to meet itself to form a circle. Unlike the Hollywood model, this implies a lateral model, not exclusive of the linear but containing it, wherein all phenomena, including urban warriors, arise mysteriously and return to their origins or source a little further on down the path, in an easy, circular manner.

Hollywoodism on the other hand implies an end to the game when the final credits scroll up on the screen.

But there is no end. When you die, the energy and consciousness generated during your lifetime here will not be destroyed. Energy and consciousness cannot be destroyed. They can only be transformed. The essence of what you've grown accustomed to thinking of as 'you' during this lifetime has always and will always exist in one dimension or another. Perhaps not in the form you've grown to recognize, but it will exist. Perhaps as an alien plant or giraffe even – it doesn't matter, you'll make the best of it at the time.

I don't want to get into talking about death just yet, I just wish to declare an end to ends. Hereafter let ends be banished and the idea of transformation take their place.

There is no goal, except perhaps to persuade yourself to be fully present in this moment, moment to moment from now on and thus reap the rewards of this universe, which after all will only ever have existence in this moment and not at some projected future date of your imagination.

The essential quality, however, of your experience in this moment or any other is entirely up to you.

Don't measure the success of your life by the goals you achieve, but by the essential quality of your experience this very moment – the quality of internal conditions in other words. This quality will be reflected automatically in external conditions (in the course of time).

In fact, why measure your life at all? Why not simply enjoy it? And to help you do so more profoundly, for surely there is nothing more important than your profound enjoyment of life, let awareness return to your body in preparation for a second tour of your internal somatic architecture. We need to install your own personal dream-essence actualization program.

INTRODUCING THE CORRECT ESSENCES FOR PERFECT DREAM ACTUALIZATION INTO YOUR INTERNAL META-NETWORK – COMMANDING YOUR ENERGY

The purpose of the following is to help you discover your true nature, not your local, so-called human nature, which is necessarily corrupted by fear and greed, but that aspect of you synonymous with the Tao. And to prepare the most favorable conditions for your true nature to flourish while you still have a body, in order that maximum enjoyment (freedom from pain) may be your lot and the lot of all with whom you interact from now on.

Only practice this if you want radical positive change in your life, because it works. If you think there's a chance you may be happier with your pain and would prefer things to remain as they are, however unsatisfactory that might be, then stop immediately.

Adjust your mainframe for optimum vertical and horizontal expansion, allowing all your muscles to relax and sink, and regulate your breathing for maximum fluidity, slowness of tempo and depth.

Situate yourself properly in triplicate simultaneously in all three inner chambers, observing from the upper, feeling from the middle and driving the experience from the lower.

Inhale. As you do so, become aware of your chattering mind. Exhale. As you do so, send the breath in a stream to your perineum (between your legs). Obviously the physical breath is not actually reaching your perineum, bound as it is within your lungs (unless, that is, you have an extraordinarily low-slung pair of lungs). This style of breathing, in fact, where you imagine sending your breath beyond its physical bounds, is called subtle breathing and is a device for helping your mind direct energy to any part of your body at will. Though the actual passage of breath is imaginary, the actual movement of energy is real.

As the subtle breath streams down to your perineum, in benign dictator mode, silently say (to your chattering mind), firmly but with compassion, 'Silence!' For as you command so shall it be. And if you find that far-fetched in these Prozac-riven times, remember this is your internal kingdom or queendom and you're the only 'one' in charge – no one and nothing else. And if your mind isn't going to listen to you, who will it listen to! Me! Yes, who! (There's more to that question than meets the eye.)

As you say the word 'silence', see the word, hear the subtle sound of the word, feel the essence of its meaning in your perineum and let 'silence' be your internal mode. Let silence fill you internally. (As far as achieving external silence these days, find a deep cave, build a soundproofed chamber, buy incredibly well-fitting earplugs or forget it.)

Inhale. As you do so, send the subtle breath in a fine stream up your super-conduit of maximum upward thrust, from your perineum up the rear face of your backbone, through the back of your neck, over the top of your brain and into the roof of your mouth.

As you do so, silently say the word 'Power!' See the word, hear its sound and feel the essence of its meaning throughout the length of the conduit. Let 'power' be your internal mode. Let power fill you internally.

Exhale. As you do so, send the subtle breath in a fine stream from above the roof of your mouth through your super-conduit of maximum downward drop back to your perineum, via the back of your throat, chest, abdomen and pubic bone.

As the subtle breath streams down to your perineum, silently say, 'Peace!' See the word, hear its sound and feel the essence of its meaning running the length of the conduit. Let peace be your internal mode. Let peace fill you internally.

Inhale. As you do so, draw the subtle breath in a fine stream from your perineum back up your super-conduit of maximum downward drop (the wrong way up the down escalator) to that point 2 inches below your navel, where it intersects your horizontal belt channel. Here the subtle breath divides into two streams, each running round your belt channel in opposite directions until meeting your upward thrust regulator channel 2 inches either side of your spine, where it streams up bilaterally in an outwardly diagonal direction like the rear section of a pair of braces (pant-suspenders) to the tips of your shoulders.

As the subtle breath streams up to your waist and around your horizontal belt channel, silently say, 'Health!' As it continues up to your shoulder-tips, silently say, 'Healing Power!' seeing the words, hearing their sound and feeling the essence of their meaning respectively along the relevant length of the route. Let health and healing (of self and potentially others) be your mode. Let health and healing fill you internally.

Exhale. As you do so send the subtle breath in a fine stream bilaterally from your shoulder-tips down the outside of your arms through your upward thrust regulator channel to the ends of your second fingers and back into the center of each palm.

As the subtle breath streams into your palms, silently say, 'Protection!' seeing the word, hearing its sound and feeling the essence of its meaning all along the length of the route. Let protection from harm be your internal mode. Let protection from harm fill you (and surround you) internally.

Inhale. As you do so, draw the subtle breath in your palms in a fine stream bilaterally up the inside of your arms through your downward drop regulator channel into your armpits. As it streams, silently say, 'Love!', seeing the word, hearing its sound and feeling the essence of its meaning all along the length of the route. Let love be your internal mode. Let love fill you internally. Let your body resonate with love.

Exhale. As you do so, send the subtle breath in your armpits in a subtle stream bilaterally down through the downward drop regulator channel, running like the front section of a pair of braces, diagonally inwards down to intersect your horizontal belt channel 2 inches either side of the mid-line at that point 2 inches below your navel. Here the subtle breath circles round to the back in opposite directions, to meet your super-conduit of maximum upward thrust at your spine where it reforms as a single stream and continues down (the wrong way on the up escalator) to your perineum.

As the subtle breath streams bilaterally down to waist level and round your horizontal belt channel to your spine, silently say 'Purity!' and as it continues down into your perineum, say, 'Beauty!', seeing the words, hearing their sound and feeling the essence of their meaning respectively run the relevant length of the route. Let purity and beauty be your inner mode. Let purity and beauty fill you internally. Let your body resonate with purity and beauty.

Inhale. As you do so, draw the subtle breath in your perineum up through your penetrating channel, along the front face of your backbone to the level of your solar plexus (upper abdomen). As the subtle breath streams up to navel level, silently say, 'Core Strength!' As it continues up to solar plexus level, say, 'Longevity!'

See the words, hear their sound and feel the essence of their meaning respectively along the relevant sections of your penetrating channel. Let core strength and longevity be your inner mode. Let core strength and longevity fill you internally till your body resonates.

Exhale. As you do so, send the subtle breath in your solar plexus back down through your penetrating channel to your perineum. Here it enters your downward drop regulator channel and divides into two streams running bilaterally along the groove between upper thigh and torso (the inguinal canal) to your outer hip joints and down the outside of your legs to the ends of your second toes and back into the balls of your feet.

As the subtle breath streams down your penetrating channel from solar plexus to perineum, silently say, 'Stamina!'

As it streams bilaterally to your outer hip joints, say, 'Endurance!' As it streams from your hips to the outside of your knees, say, 'Steadfastness!'

And as it streams from your knees down to the balls of your feet, say, 'Sturdiness!'

See the words, hear their sound and feel the essence of their meaning respectively along the relevant sections of the route. Let stamina, endurance, steadfastness and sturdiness be your inner mode. Let yourself be internally filled with stamina, endurance, steadfastness and sturdiness. Let your body resonate with their essence.

Inhale. As you do so, draw the subtle breath through your upward thrust regulator channel running from the balls of your feet in a fine stream, bilaterally back along the instep of each foot, under the inner ankle joints, up the inside of each leg and into the perineum. There the two streams unite and continue up (the down escalator) your super-conduit of maximum downward drop to that point 2 inches below your navel.

As the subtle breath streams upwards from the balls of your feet to the inside of your knees, silently say, 'Confidence!'

As it continues up the inside of your thighs to your perineum, say, 'Motivation!'

As it continues up from your perineum to that point 2 inches below your navel, say, Trust!' See the words, hear their sound and feel the essence of their meaning respectively resonate along the relevant sections of the route.

Let confidence, motivation and trust be your inner mode. Let yourself be filled internally with confidence, motivation and trust.

Exhale. As you do so, send the subtle breath from that point 2 inches below your navel back down your super-conduit of maximum downward drop into your perineum. As the subtle breath streams into your perineum, say, 'Integrity!', seeing the word, hearing its sound and feeling the essence of its meaning resonate along the route. Let integrity be your inner mode. Let the essence of integrity fill you internally.

Inhale. Draw the subtle breath back up your super-conduit of maximum upward thrust again from your perineum up over your brain to the roof of your mouth, saying, 'Power!', placing and experiencing the essence of the word appropriately (you know the score by now).

Exhale. Send the subtle breath from the roof of your mouth back down the front of your body to your perineum through your super-conduit of maximum downward drop, saying, 'Peace!' (OK!)

Inhale. Draw the subtle breath in your perineum up your super-conduit of maximum downward drop to that point 2 inches below your navel. As you do so, say, 'Abundance!', projecting the word visually and sonically along that section of the conduit and letting your body resonate with the essence of its meaning. Let abundance be your inner mode. Let abundance fill you internally (if you wish it to fill you externally).

Exhale. As you do so, send the subtle breath back down the conduit into your perineum to join your downward drop regulator channel wherein it forks outwards along the inguinal canals to your outer hip joints and streams down the outside of your legs to your second toes and back into the balls of your feet.

As it passes your perineum, say, 'Success!' and feel your whole body, from the perineum outwards, resonate with it.

As the subtle breath streams from your perineum into the balls of your feet, say, 'Magnetism!', projecting the word visually and sonically along the length of the route, and letting its essence resonate throughout.

Inhale. As you do so, draw the subtle breath into the balls of your feet up along the inside of your legs through your upward thrust regulator channel to your perineum and from your perineum into your genital channel to the tip of your uterus or penis (depending on which one you 'own').

As the subtle breath reaches the penile or uterine tip, say, 'Sensuality!', or 'Sexuality!' if you prefer, projecting the word visually and sonically along the length of the route, allowing your body to resonate with the essence of its meaning from the genitals out.

Exhale. As you do so, send the subtle breath from the penile or uterine tip along the return genital channel back into your perineum. As it streams back into your perineum, say 'Honor!' projecting the word appropriately. Let honor be your internal mode (and thus guide your external actions). This is important because by this stage the subtle breath has stirred your generative fires giving rise to a probable increase in your personal sexual power (in relation to others). In any case, it is preferable to contain the generative fire now as you are about to transmute it first into chi in your lower chamber, then into 'soul' or individuated spirit in your middle chamber, and finally into universal spirit or Tao in your upper chamber via the following.

Inhale. As you do so, draw the subtle breath from your perineum up along the front face of your backbone through your penetrating channel once more to the level of that point 2 inches below your navel, where it now enters your lower chamber (through the back door). As it does, say, 'Limitless Power!'. See the words. Hear their sound. Feel the essence of their meaning reverberate within your lower chamber and radiate outwards to resonate throughout your entire being.

Exhale. As you do so, draw the subtle breath from your lower chamber out through the back door and upwards along your penetrating channel to the level of the chest where it enters your middle chamber through the back door.

As the subtle breath streams into your middle chamber, say, 'Absolute Harmony!', seeing the words, hearing their sound and feeling the essence of their meaning resound in your middle chamber and vibrate in waves radiating to all parts of your being (and beyond).

Inhale. As you do so, draw the subtle breath in your middle chamber out through the back door and up through your penetrating channel to your upper chamber in the center of your brain where it enters through the back door in your upper brainstem.

As the subtle breath streams into your upper chamber, say, 'Eternal Duration!', seeing the words, hearing their sound and feeling the essence of their meaning reverberate inside your skull (for ever and ever) and radiating outwards to resonate with your entire energy field (for miles around).

In the midst of this resonance, exhale, and as you do so, send the subtle breath from your upper chamber, out of the back door and down your penetrating channel again to your perineum.

As the subtle breath streams back into your perineum, still in the midst of the resonance of 'eternal duration', say, 'Immortal Spirit Body!' and in this precise moment you are that and may experience yourself (momentarily) unbounded by physical form. You will (momentarily) feel larger than your mainframe and are able, if you want, to amplify this state to universal proportions – become limitless, omnipresent and synonymous with your true nature, the Tao, in other words.

Thus identified, inhale and draw what is now the subtle breath of the entire Tao from your perineum, up your super-conduit of upward maximum thrust to that point in the center of the base of your skull where flesh meets bone (the 'eye' or 'opening' at the back of your head through which cosmic intelligence enters your mainframe).

As the subtle breath streams into this point, say, 'Creativity!', seeing the word, hearing its sound and feeling the essence of its meaning reverberate and fill not only your internal being, but the entire universe within you.

Exhale. As you do so, send the subtle breath at the base of your skull over the top of your brain along your super-conduit of maximum upward thrust to that point in the middle of your forehead just above the bridge of your nose

As the subtle breath streams into this point, say, 'Manifestation!', seeing the word, hearing its sound and feeling the essence and full implication of its meaning reverberate in the center of your forehead and radiate outwards endlessly.

Exhale. As you do so, send the subtle breath in the center of your forehead down through the roof of your mouth into your super-conduit of maximum downward drop and back down to your perineum, which is now the 'gate of mortality' of the entire universe.

Remain in this state, breathing gently and slowly, while you integrate the experience and finally allow the subtle breath in your perineum to permeate your bones to be stored for further use.

So now you see why the body is your temple. But as Raja Ram said, it's a nightclub too, so how can you have some fun with this new-found friend, your immortal spirit body?

YOU AND YOUR IMMORTAL SPIRIT BODY

The thing about suddenly realizing you have a spirit body is not to make a big deal about it. In a multidimensional quantum universe like this it's a perfectly ordinary phenomenon.

It may seem odd or bizarre to even entertain such ideas. But that's to be expected when looking from the perspective of your previous self in the four-dimensional world.

But now, having pushed aside the veil with which you had hitherto obscured the fifth dimension, it becomes no more extraordinary than, say, the introduction of mobile video phones. You always knew there was someone behind that voice. Now you can see them too. So what? After the initial curiosity and excitement has worn off, which in these days of high-speed information bombardment happens all too rapidly, it becomes commonplace. This doesn't mean you don't value the facility itself; you just don't let the excitement of its novelty value ruffle your feathers.

If you get too agitated about it, your spirit body will vanish, or at least your awareness of it will, until you calm down and reassemble yourself appropriately.

This is not meant to imply fragility on the part of your spirit body, which, being ever present, everlasting and optionally expandable to all-encompassing, is intrinsically indestructible. And it's not me telling you that. You just ordained it to be so during the previously guided internal tour (de force).

Remember, according to both the Taoists and Einsteins of this world, all reality is subjective, or rather all realities are subjective. Hence, as you ordain (command), so shall it be. This is even and especially true when effecting multidimensional quantum change in the very fabric of (your subjective) reality.

But as I say, it's a subtle process you're immersed in here, which requires much sensitivity on your part. You are not, after all, attempting to leave dimensions one to four to exist in the fifth dimension or beyond. Leave that till you die. You are merely expanding inner awareness exponentially until it becomes multidimensional. Thus your awareness simultaneously spans both the visible world of form and appearance and the invisible world from which that springs.

To attempt this without being first properly internally assembled is to invite the onset of symptoms normally associated with paranoid schizophrenia. Without proper self-placement within your internal somatic architecture it is impossible to achieve the required balance and you will fall prey to delusions. Which is why you need to return (in triplicate) to your trio of inner chambers frequently throughout the day, if only for mere nanoseconds, even (and especially) while otherwise externally engaged in the business of negotiating the details of workaday urban life.

Not just to prevent the onset of madness, of course, but more importantly to nurture this fledgling relationship with your own immortal self.

Talking of multidimensional relationships, with all this emphasis on personal inner-awakening it would be mistaken of you to imagine this to be merely a self-absorbed solo adventure. On the contrary, you may find it comforting to embrace the following.

YOU ARE NOT ALONE

To fully appreciate this, check your mainframe for maximum vertical and horizontal expansion, relax and sink your muscles, regulate your breathing for optimum fluidity, evenness and depth and reassemble yourself appropriately in triplicate in your trio of inner chambers, witnessing from the upper, feeling from the middle and driving from the lower – observe the familiar protocol in other words.

From your vantage point in your upper chamber, picture a web of intersecting fibers similar in etheric composition to your own internal energy super-conduits, originating in your lower chamber, stretched out omnidirectionally on the horizontal plane and extending to infinity.

In all directions on the horizontal, as far as the inner eye can see (on the screen on the back of the forehead in front of you, or stowed in your armrest in business and first), is an endless field of crisscrossing fibers forming points of intersection, one of which happens to be bang in the middle of your lower chamber.

In fact at each point of intersection is a light glowing more or less brightly. Each (point of) light is an individuated collection point of consciousness, a spirit or 'soul', as are you.

As in your own case, the more awake the individuated spirit, the brighter burns their light.

This infinite sea of lights exists in the fifth dimension and therefore traverses all boundaries of time and space (even though your personal point of access is within your physical mainframe, which owes its material existence very much to dimensions one, two, three and four).

Thus you are connected by a point in your lower chamber, in the same place as your small intestine, to every conscious being throughout the entire universe. As this connective web is interdimensionally ubiquitous and therefore unbounded by the normal operating rules of time and space (dimensions one through four), this means a potential telepathic connection with everyone who has ever lived, is living now and will ever live (in the future).

Talk of rolling a product out to a broader market. Can you imagine the potential marketing opportunity here? We're talking direct telepathic viral marketing.

But that notwithstanding, ponder for a moment on the enormity of this picture and its implications.

Imagine being able to connect energetically your consciousness with the consciousness of everyone who has ever lived, is living and will live – not just humans but all manner of life forms, alien or otherwise, even including 'angels' and other intelligence beyond the realms of imagination.

Imagine the quality and depth of information you'd be privy to if you could connect directly and instantaneously through the web to all the brightest lights in the universe throughout all time and space.

Imagine not only the quality of help and guidance you could receive from such august etheric company but also how beneficially you could affect the consciousness of everyone else with your own brand of etheric cheer.

Imagine having that crew as your invisible allies as you wander down the great thoroughfare of daily street life.

Now, to make your head really spin with the full impact of how etherically not alone you actually are, imagine this two-dimensional horizontal web becoming three dimensional, i.e. with height and depth as well. Now you can see an infinite number of points of light extending endlessly in all directions simultaneously, not just around you but above and below you too – forever and ever. Next to this the internet is a flint tool in comparison.

In effect, this web is none other than the connective consciousness of existence, the Tao, and all the individuated points of light merely different positions through which the Tao or God (there, I said it again) can experience itself, thus gaining an infinite number of differing perspectives simultaneously. So if you've ever wondered how that God of the old school was always able to know everything about everybody all the time, you need wonder no longer. It's through the etheric web that the 'one' becomes many and the many become 'one'.

But the etheric web is not just all about playing God.

On a less grandiose scale, it is possible to log on any time of day or night (and it only takes a nanosecond) to ask for help in moment-to-moment situations no matter what and, as sure as cosmic eggs is cosmic eggs, help will come on the ground in real time.

The more awake you are (the more appropriately internally arranged that is), the brighter shines your etheric point of light, and the more you get noticed. (This extends to life in dimensions one through four as well.) Which means that help, in the form of energy, ideas and even so-called miracles or unexplainable quantum events, will find you more easily.

By the same token, you are able to send help or energy to other points of light. Life is not a one-way street. You receive proportionately to what you give, whether on the street in real time or in the ether.

In this regard, as you sit internally gazing out at the web from your upper chamber, let the first thing you do be to cause the essence of peace, healing, abundance and love to emanate from you omnidirectionally and multidimensionally throughout the etheric web to be received by all who need it. This can be effected by silently commanding, 'Emanate!', seeing the word, hearing its sound and feeling the essence of its meaning reverberate in your trio of inner chambers, while visualizing, if you want, the essence of your emanation entering the fibers of the web at the point of intersection in your lower chamber.

It's like buying your ticket it puts you in credit. Though it is obviously a sign of internal development (as a warrior) when you find yourself emanating just for the hell of it and not for the pay-off, it doesn't matter if your motivation for emanating is purely selfish. As long as you emanate. This applies to life in dimensions one through four as well of course. In fact, a by-product of emanating etherically like this in the fifth dimension is a spontaneous increase in emanation levels on the bioplasmic plane too, making you a veritable powerhouse of radiant charisma as you strut your urban-warrior stuff on the street.

By the immutable laws of cause and effect and through the agency of synergy, the essence you emanate returns to you exponentially multiplied (in this instant by the number of recipients).

Consequently, once the proactive emanating phase completes itself (once, in other words, you sense your emanations have been received), make yourself switch from proactive to receptive mode, by silently issuing the command 'Receive!', while observing the usual command protocol.

Now, momentarily empty (of desire), allow yourself the luxury of watching the essence of peace, healing, abundance and love bounce back at you, exponentially multiplied, along the fibers of the etheric web, from all directions (time and dimensions) at once. Receive it into your lower chamber and let it rise up through your penetrating channel into your middle and upper chambers to reverberate throughout your spirit body (and physical mainframe).

Remember to (silently) say, Thank you!' (Always remember to say thank you – the heartfelt expression of gratitude sets up a field of harmonic resonance that keeps your spirit body and by extension your physical mainframe automatically attracting positive emanations through the web even when offline.)

(Thank you.)

In practice (and with practice), this whole procedure can be performed in the twinkling of an inner eye and need not cut brusquely into your agenda. However only practice repeatedly if you really do want increase your worldly success (among other benefits), as what you are actually effecting here is a handle on the very mechanics of good fortune or so-called divine providence itself. (Which as you know, is always good for business.)

FALLING BACKWARDS

Implicit in the super-charged tempo of post-modern, high-speed urbanized reality, when seen in context of the past-present-future progression of linear time within whose confines we appear to live out our daily four-dimensional existence, is an incessant drive forwards into the (projected) future, as if our salvation lies there. As if liberation – freedom from pain, suffering and restriction – exists only in the future. As if when you've made enough money to buy your subtropical hideaway, have your breasts enlarged, support the perfect lover, or employ a personal assistant to field your emails, phone calls and text messages and to pick up your dry cleaning, for example, you will at last attain salvation.

No need to rehash that same old spiritual dogma here, where I tell you that salvation – liberation from pain, suffering and restriction – does not come at some (projected) point in the future, nor at the hands of another human being, nor even in material acquisitions (though the PA would be a help).

No need to pound the point into the ground telling you that true liberation is only available here and now, this very moment (and of course during the here and now of every subsequent moment between this one and the moment of death).

No need to use this opportunity to exhort or cajole you into remembering to go within for your salvation, nor indeed induce you to partake of any such 'spiritual7 clichés.

There exists a whole raft of self-help books far more eloquent and erudite than this humble pile of words from which such perennial advice (and faux-spiritual propaganda) can be gleaned. And in any case, I'm sure by now you already know.

I won't even take this opportunity to say that if you want to survive this high-speed lifestyle intact, you must take time out each day to simply 'stop'. For as wise as that advice would appear, it is in fact impossible to achieve.

Everything in the entirety of existence is in motion. A fundamental quality of existence is, in fact, perpetual motion.

Within the bounds of four-dimensional reality, caught as you apparently are in the progression of linear time, you cannot stop. You either go forwards or you go backwards. In the world of perpetual motion there is no in-between.

Furthermore, according to the end-game Hollywood model, to fall backwards at this point in the game implies falling away from reaching your temporal goals, losing your place in the race and surrendering to entropic tendencies. Like the plane you're on going into reverse in mid-air, while on a transatlantic night flight over the wastes of Greenland during an electric storm in the dread cold of winter (I know I keep mentioning it, but am I the only one who has had to repeatedly endure that horror or am I just developing long-haul flight phobia?) the idea of falling backwards fills us with horror.

Instinctively we want only forward momentum. You can test this by standing with feet together with a sturdy catching partner three or so feet behind you and allowing your body to fall back into their waiting arms without moving your feet from their original position on the floor. You will find it requires courage (and someone who knows how to catch you properly).

So we don't like falling backwards. That is until we get used to it and realize that, all along, it was one of life's greatest pleasures.

The Taoists in fact knew this all along. What lies behind you in fact is often far more relevant to your healthy growth than what lies before (you).

Much mention, in fact, is made by competent instructors of both Taoist martial arts and meditation of the importance of developing awareness at the back of your head (at that point at the skull's base where bone meets flesh) to what's going on behind you (both physically and metaphorically). They will instruct you to practice walking around with that point 'open' like a rear eye or rear view mirror through which you can 'see', 'hear' or develop awareness of what's going on behind you in order specifically to complete and fortify your protective energy shield (to be explained later).

However, the Taoists noticed that if one observed the usual protocol (eyes shut, physical mainframe at maximum vertical and horizontal expansion, muscles sunk in full relaxation, breathing at optimum fluidity, evenness and depth, with awareness assembled appropriately in triplicate within one's trio of inner chambers one could enjoy the indescribable inner thrill of falling backwards in inner space at unimaginable speeds. They discovered (in accordance with the immutable laws of yin and yang and things not always being as they appear) that far from leading to entropy or dissolution, surrendering to the backward 'flow', as they called it, would in fact not only take one back to the very source of life itself, the Tao, but would actually enhance your forward momentum in relation to achievement of material goals. They found that, by allowing oneself to literally fall back into the source, one would become so recharged with profound energy and insight that when one returned to normal waking state and the details of daily life, one would be hardly able to contain oneself, so damn good would one feel (in every possible way, on every possible level, about every possible thing).

They also found that the increase in chi regular backward falling produced would help one live a longer, healthier life.

Moreover, and most importantly, they discovered that with each successive backward flight, one would become progressively more liberated from pain, suffering and restriction (both on the inner and outer strata of reality).

Could falling backwards, then, be the key to personal freedom, when all along you thought it was springing forward? Could those old Taoists have been right?

Moreover, could they have been right when they pointed out that if one conducted such internal backward flight, while consciously in spirit-body mode on account of having paid adequate prior attention to all aforementioned spirit-body identity development procedures, one would gain such personal power in so flying, one would want to run down the street shouting 'Halleluiah, I now know the very secrets of existence itself!' if one wasn't such a self- contained urban warrior in the Taoist mold?

Could they have been right to point out that regularly thus flying, one would, by returning to the source, be in some way actually travelling backwards through time, in some way reversing the clock and very passage of years themselves, and in so doing actually start looking progressively physically younger, less lined and altogether more radiant and beautiful? Could they be right to consider such flights of the spirit body tantamount to availing oneself of the very elixir of eternal youth (and immortality)?

Personally, I can tell you they were. And if you don't believe me, just look at the author's photographic likeness and you'll have to admit I don't look half bad for someone of 93.

However, don't take my word for it. Be like the old Taoists and try it for yourself, but only if you want to increase personal power levels, universal insight, life span, general charisma, physical strength and beauty, relaxation levels and material success.

If so, adjust mainframe for maximum vertical and horizontal expansion (repetition of fundamental instructions still deliberate, by the way), muscles for full sinking and relaxation and breathing for optimum fluidity, evenness and depth of origin.

Assemble yourself in triplicate within your trio of inner chambers (witnessing from the upper, feeling from the middle and driving from the lower).

Inhale. As you do so, draw the subtle breath from your perineum through your super-conduit of maximum upward thrust over the top of your brain into the area just above the roof of your mouth.

Exhale. As you do so, send the subtle breath back down to your perineum through your super-conduit of maximum downward drop to complete the loop.

This is the minimum amount of super-channel activation necessary to safeguard integrity of your etheric shape as you fly – to prevent possible psychic disintegration in other words, in cases of recent or latent mental instability. However, don't resist the urge to complete a full tour of your internal somatic architecture at this point, if the urge should arise.

In any case, once you've completed at least one satisfactory loop and the subtle breath and awareness has returned to your perineum, silently say, 'Spirit Body!' See the words, hear their sound and feel the essence of their meaning reverberate in your perineum, those reverberations radiating outwards to find resonance throughout your mainframe, and allow yourself a moment's identification with the object of your summons, your spirit body.

Thus identified, and hence momentarily unbounded by the constraints of your physical mainframe, allow yourself to fall backwards (through the back of your head), and just keep falling. As you fall (backwards and backwards), allow yourself to pick up speed, accelerating until you feel as if you're falling faster than even the speed of light itself.

Keep some awareness of the physical rudiments (mainframe expansion, relaxation and breathing), because though this experience is occurring in the fifth dimension, it is facilitated by the body and will be much smoother and more substantial when the body and therefore energy flow is appropriately adjusted.

There will come a point in the falling that, as your speed reaches the point of critical mass, you will feel as if you come to a still point of no momentum.

Simultaneously, you will feel a presence behind you, supporting you in deepest darkest inner space, into which you seem to have reversed yourself and which on closer inspection reveals itself to be none other than you yourself – Big You, your true nature, the Tao in other words, who seems to have been waiting patiently all these aeons for you to return (to yourself).

Welcome home.

When you feel instinctively that you've spent enough time at source luxuriating in the 'warm waters of true nature', in your spiritual bubble bath – and it only requires less than a nanosecond to be of impact – simply open your eyes.

There is no need to elaborate a forward journey to bring you back into the present moment, unless inclined towards making drama where none is required, as you will never be more in the moment than this.

Simply open your eyes while gently retaining perspective from the depths of inner space and carry on as you were.

In fact, in practice and with practice you will be able, as were those Taoists of old, to effect an instantaneous backward flight with eyes wide open while otherwise engaged in the details of daily (or nightly) life, whether at work, rest or play. Remember, it all happens in the fifth dimension, outside the bounds of linear time (and space).

I realize I could have simply conveyed all the above with a complete absence of ceremony, by simply saying, 'Close your eyes and fall backwards through inner space!'; but I felt that such a precious jewel as this was worthy of the preceding fanfare, lest it got inadvertently overlooked in the rush (through your agenda).

However, if I were simply to say, 'Close your eyes and fall backwards through inner space!' you'd know exactly what to do now. (Wouldn't you!)

SELF-PROTECTION AND PROTECTION OF OTHERS

As previously mentioned, there will be times when, on account of being momentarily distracted by the pull of greed, lust, anger (intolerance), doubt, vanity, sloth or envy, you will find yourself internally disassembled, physically disheveled or both, during which awareness of your spirit body will recede, rendering you vulnerable to the negative energy of others. Others who sometimes may be quite twisted and who may express their twist as a form of attack upon your person, whether psychic or indeed physical.

At such times, it will beneficial for you to effect 'erection' of a protective energy shield.

It is the erection of such a shield that lies at the heart of all martial art practice – training of skills in the physical combat aspect being merely a metaphor for developing an impenetrable psychic shield. Not that developing actual combat skills isn't worthwhile. On the contrary; but as any accomplished martial artist well-versed in combat skills will tell you, if you arrive at the point during an untoward exchange with someone when you actually employ those combat skills, something must have gone seriously wrong with your training. It would indicate a breach in your psychic shield, which had allowed the negative energy of the 'opponent' to find resonance within your own internal somatic architecture, thus leaving you vulnerable to violence. (Big mistake.)

Obviously at times like these, the martial artist would be glad of his or her combat skills. My teacher of combat arts once said to me (as his parting shot just before leaving town for good and after months of often brutal training, during which I'd learned to ward off all manner of vicious attack),'So you wanna learn self-defense?' 1 responded bemused and slightly hesitant, as always when faced with his enigmatic riddles, 'Er yes'. 'Then go and buy a gun!' at which he turned and walked off into the New Mexican sunset never to be heard of again.

In other words, no matter how well trained you happen to be in combat skills, you don't stand much chance against a gun – there'll always be someone better tooled-up than you, one way or another.

The trick is to deflect negative energy long before it manifests as a physical threat to your person. Because as any urban warrior knows, violence is to be avoided at all costs (wherever humanly possible).

To which end you might do as the Taoist martial arts master, avail yourself of the following facility. This will enable you to erect an effective psychic shield of protective energy capable of deflecting all incoming negative energy whether expressed physically, psychically or even economically, and so evermore walk the great thoroughfare in peace and safety.

Attend to the basic preliminaries, adjusting your physical mainframe, muscles and breathing appropriately and internally assembling yourself properly within your three inner chambers.

Inhale.

Exhale. As you do so, let this cause the subtle breath to collect in your perineum.

Inhale. As you do so, draw the subtle breath backwards and up the rear face of your backbone through your super-conduit of maximum upward thrust to the level of a point on your spine, itself on the same level as that point 2 inches below your navel (at the upper reaches of your lower back just above the level of your waist in other words), where your super-conduit of maximum upward thrust intersects your horizontal belt channel.

Exhale. As you do so, send the subtle breath around your horizontal belt channel in two streams each moving outwards and round to the front, one to the left and one to the right, till they meet at that point 2 inches below your navel, ready to cross (over each other).

Inhale. As you do so, propel each stream further round the belt channel till they both meet and cross again at the previous point on your backbone.

Exhale as they cross, and move back round to your front again and so on, causing these two streams of subtle breath to perpetuate their motion round your horizontal belt channel in opposing directions, propelled by your inhalation and exhalation.

Keep breathing, using your breath as a pump to propel the motion of subtle breath and gradually notice the subtle breath accelerate until moving at the speed of light and beyond.

Now picture this. Each of these two rings, spinning in opposing directions round your horizontal belt channel, are in fact each at the center of a giant spinning sphere of energy of approximately 9 feet in diameter, extending naturally above and beneath you as well as around you.

These two spheres each spinning at the speed of light or more in opposing directions, are concentric and therefore coexist spatially with you and specifically your lower chamber at their joint center.

If you find that a difficult vision to hold for an appreciable length of time, imagine the energy comprising them as two different shades of brightly colored light. If you like, make the one spinning leftwards light green and the one spinning rightwards light blue. It doesn't matter – in this instant you are merely employing these colors as a device to aid visualization and need not concern yourself with their significance. Light green and blue are fairly neutral in the scale of color, easy to 'see' and their effects generally cleansing and healing and so safe to use for these purposes.

Obviously the darker the shade employed, the more potentially agitating, and thus only suitable for experimentation by one more conversant with the technique. There's a risk of self-contamination by, say, crimson or black light, which though tending to have a more noticeably potent effect when employed against an 'opponent's' attack can also more easily backfire on you in cases where your 'opponent's' energy field is stronger – it does happen from time to time. So stick to the light greens and blues for the time being at least.

Having activated these spheres, you may simply leave them spinning while you carry on as you were, returning to attend to spin maintenance with enough regularity that, if called upon to use the psychic shield they provide in public, you'll be able to do so without a moment's hesitation.

This applies to all time spent in the company of others where negative energy is or may be present. Even when simply walking past someone in the street with a preponderance of negative energy where you get that subtle feeling of disgust that makes you not want to breathe in as they pass. (In fact, at such times it is better to exhale as if passing by a bad smell, to prevent unconsciously 'breathing 'their negativity into you.) In order to help diffuse any potential internal agitation, which may hinder your instantaneous self-assemblage when dealing with the hostility of others or merely a mild distaste arising from the briefest encounter, you should bear the following suggestion firmly in mind at all times.

DON'T TAKE IT PERSONALLY

No matter how much it appears otherwise, someone else's hostility towards you, in whatever form that hostility is expressed in your direction, is not actually personal.

Everyone on this planet, however it may appear otherwise to you, is actually doing the best they can according to their current state of personal development. This applies even to the most twisted people you can think of.

Everyone is doing the very best they can relative to their current personal state of evolution, governed by variables too numerous to quantify, but which include environmental, social, geographical, political, gender-related, cultural, genetic, constitutional factors in relation to that person's conditions of upbringing, as well as more esoteric factors including results of past life cause and effect.

This applies equally to you as to others.

This is not to condone twisted behavior, thoughts and actions, but merely to point out that, were we not all doing the very best we can, each according to our particular stage of inner development, things would be in far more of a conundrum out on the street than they already are (if such a state of affairs can be imagined).

Naturally, what we are concerned with in this book is the acceleration of personal growth, not just for your own benefit, but for the greater benefit of everyone with whom you interact, which potentially means everyone. Every warrior, indeed every Buddha, knows that not a single one of us (in the entire universe) can be fully liberated (from pain, suffering and restriction) until we all are.

By the same token, if only one of us manages full liberation, we all will.

The anticipated acceleration of inner self-development, therefore, is required (from the collective perspective) to accelerate the onset of liberation of us all, no matter the extent of our individual twistedness and how that may be expressed as hostility or just plain smelliness towards your person.

It's not personal, but that doesn't mean you must leave yourself vulnerable to it. That's where discernment comes into it with regards to deciphering the difference between negative and positive energy. But discernment arises naturally as soon as you are properly assembled internally, through agency of your middle chamber, which gives you the ability to feel, or be sensitive to what's going on within in response to external conditions.

With discernment and the facility of an active sheath of protective energy, you will be fully protected from harm from now on. Providing of course, you ensure you stand in good relation to your world and everyone in it. (And that means me too, baby, so pay attention.)

STANDING IN GOOD RELATION TO YOUR WORLD AND EVERYONE IN IT (INCLUDING ME)

Even in context of the four-dimensional phantasmagorical conundrum we usually refer to as 'real life', where money and social status are the standard criteria by which individuals' worth is evaluated, the qualities of kindness and generosity (of spirit as well as material wealth) still earn you more respect in the long run.

Why would this be so?

Because even in such a confused milieu as this current global society – comprised as it is of a species (apparently) in its death throes, no longer facing the prospect but the reality of overcrowding (of land, sea, air and even space), rapidly dwindling essential resources (both for sustenance and prevention of endemic disease), accelerating breakdown of law and order, growing entrenchment of corruption, and swiftly rising levels of sheer stupidity exhibited on a global level by the so-called leaders of the world's great nations (wherein a far greater proportion of public energy is directed to the cult of celebrity worship and daily engrossment in third rate soap operas than in attempting to discover ways round the crisis threatening our very immediate collective survival)—even in such a mishmashed milieu as this, we all fundamentally still value one 'thing' above all others: love.

Even if it's completely unconscious. Even if we misguidedly seek it through fame, fortune, temporal power, status, gratuitous sex, the acquisition of possessions, or violence, what we are unconsciously searching for is love.

Which is why kindness and generosity – the expression of love in action, in other words – still makes you stand out in the crowd.

For after all, are not all your activities, whether in pursuit of money or fun, dependent to the greater extent on your relationships with those with whom you are required to interact in the pursuit of all your temporal goals?

When you radiate those qualities, therefore (not in a namby-pamby way that would make others take advantage of you, but in the way of the urban warrior – one who is so appropriately internally assembled as to evoke respect from all with whom he or she interacts during the course of a busy globally urbanized lifetime), when from a place of internal power you act with intrinsic kindness and generosity, not only will your innate love oil the wheels of your relationships and facilitate the actualization of temporal goals, but you will also be increasing the flow of the one 'thing' everyone, including everyone throughout the universal etheric web even as far as the god of the old-school, wants: love.

Truly there is nothing more powerful, nothing more valuable or valued (if only unconsciously).

And according to the immutable law that states that what you put out returns to you exponentially multiplied by the number of recipients, when you start emanating love, through the expression of spontaneous acts of unconditional kindness and generosity, you set up a field of harmonic resonance that will attract so much love towards you in return, you may have to sit down for a while to get your bearings.

But before you do, in connection with this theme of standing in good relation to all with whom and with which you interact, it could benefit you to pragmatically examine the following.

To institute a personal field of positive harmonic resonance that spontaneously causes you to perform acts of kindness and generosity without premeditation or contrivance – the performance of which will nonetheless attract great good fortune to your person in return, will moreover benefit and gladden the hearts of all those recipient to such acts, and will provide inspiration for onlookers to do likewise (i.e. to set up the internal conditions for you to conduct yourself as a holy man or woman while still engaged in worldly pursuits) and so automatically adjust your stance in relation to the world around you, especially when deeply identifying with your spirit body through practice of all preceding instruction – stand up.

Stand up. With feet 2 inches apart, pelvis slightly tucked under (as if in mild sexual thrust), belly relaxed, chest relaxed, back of the neck relaxed, mainframe at maximum vertical and horizontal expansion, all soft tissue fully sunk groundwards and breath at optimum fluidity, evenness and depth.

With weight evenly distributed between both feet, while tilted slightly forwards towards the balls of the feet, assemble yourself internally within your three inner chambers, witnessing from the upper, feeling from the middle and driving from the lower.

Slowly raise your arms out sideways to just above shoulder height with palms facing forwards, to form a crucifix shape. Mentally extend from your backbone through your upper back, shoulder joints, elbows, wrists and knuckles to the tips of your fingers, while not actually physically extending so much that you cause strain on the relevant muscles, tendons and ligaments. Let your bones form the shape while your muscles – especially your shoulders and neck – relax and sink.

Command your spirit body into awareness, by silently saying, 'Spirit Body!', seeing the word, hearing its sound and feeling the essence of its meaning (to you) reverberate throughout your upstanding mainframe.

Inhale. As you do so, draw the subtle breath as it from the center of the Earth, through the balls of your feet, back past your inner ankle joints and up through your upward thrust regulator channel into your perineum, up through your penetrating channel and into your lower chamber by the back door.

Simultaneously (on the same inhalation) draw another stream of subtle breath as if from heaven-central, down through the crown of your head, down through your penetrating channel and into your lower chamber by the back door (as well).

This was traditionally known as 'joining heaven and Earth' and was considered by Taoists the ancient Orient over to be your highest function as a human being on the planet. It represents the mixing of the original essences of yin and yang necessary to lend substance to any phenomenon (in this case the 'love-package' about to be emanated by you).

Exhale. As you do so, draw the subtle breath (transporting the heaven-earth, yin-yang mix) out through the back door of your inner chamber into your horizontal belt channel, which it meets on your spine and outwards 2 inches either side, to join the bilateral strands of your upward thrust regulator channel running diagonally outwardly up both sides of your back to your shoulder tips (like the rear section of a pair of braces), and along the outside of your arms to your second fingers, into the center of each palm (stigmata points) from where it emanates from your mainframe into the ether beyond.

As the mix passes either side of your middle chamber on its way bilaterally up your back let it be infused with (your) love. You may wish to command it so, by silently saying, 'Love!' as it passes by, seeing the word, hearing its sound and feeling the essence of its meaning (to you), reverberate along your arms, through your palms and beyond in the surrounding ether.

Put simply, your inhalation draws primordial energy, both from the ground below you and from the sky above simultaneously, along the vertical axis of your mainframe into your lower chamber where it forms a mix. Your (subsequent) exhalation draws that mix up past your middle chamber for a personal love-injection and outwards along the horizontal axis of your mainframe, now extended through your outstretched arms, into the surrounding ether to be made use of by all others existing on the same lateral plane as you – everyone in your world in other words.

The vertical pole of the crucifix conducts fifth-dimensional universal energy towards you, where it is enhanced with (your) love and conducted away from you through the horizontal pole to benefit your world (and the people living in it).

In this way, you institute an energetic template that will automatically subtly shift the hue and tone of your thoughts to guide your moment-to-moment actions along more compassionate lines and leave you standing in good relation to your world at all times.

Thus do you fulfil your personal messianic mission, to connect heaven and earth.

But in case messianic zeal runs away with you and lands you in the nuthouse, lower your arms slowly to your sides, luxuriating in the muscular relief, and inhale to draw subtle breath from your perineum up your super-conduit of maximum upward thrust, over your brain to the roof of your mouth. Exhale to send the subtle breath down through your super-conduit of maximum downward drop back into your perineum, thus completing a loop, in order to redefine your spirit body shape in case of energy leakages caused by over-developed messianic tendencies (latent or otherwise).

In a sense, this is like voluntarily crucifying yourself, by momentarily subjugating personal striving to the benefit of (the) all. As well as being helpful in self-development terms, this is a useful practice to prepare you for the possibility of actual crucifixion, for which, if it should transpire to be your 'end', you will be more prepared now than would have otherwise been the case.

Incidentally, before you start getting nervous, the crucifix was never trademarked by official Christianity and had a place in one form or another in the symbolism of most preconsumerist cultures, including the Taoists, the Hopis, the Ancient Egyptians and the Celts. The intersection of vertical and horizontal poles represents the individuated spirit or point of light in its 'highest' state as one who connects the fifth dimension with dimensions one through four, the yang and the yin, or heaven and Earth, in other words.

Additionally, the subtle upper body strength gained on the way will help stabilize your emotions.

Of course, on a purely physical level, the above is damn good for your cardiovascular and respiratory systems, stimulating circulation in your brachial plexii (the major nerve plexii in your armpits), and will help reduce chronic neck and shoulder tension as well as give tone to your arms. Note the feeling of blessed horizontal expansion across chest and upper back afforded you by this practice, especially on the release.

With all this talk of self-crucifixion, it would only be good manners to mention a word or two (thousand) about death, its place in the Taoist scheme of things and how it might affect you as an urban warrior, both in daily or nightly life and thereafter at the grand crossing and beyond.

THE BIG D

I doubt there's anyone alive who doesn't have some issue with the idea of their own demise. Even if you're absolutely suicidal and long for the day, it's still an issue.

Latter-day Taoist cosmology has all kinds of imagery concerning the 'afterlife' – golden immortals riding the backs of the seven celestial winds and the like. But none of them knew for sure, no matter how deeply enlightened. No one does. Not you. Not me.

It's true that by developing spirit-body awareness, you will over time generate a certain confidence about facing your own moment of death. You will also develop an instinct that your consciousness will continue, as well as a sense that at the moment of dropping your body, nothing will happen. You'll simply be where you always were, especially during such meditational moments as proposed in this book, in the fifth dimension, where time, space and form (as we know it) cease to exist. You will also find with practice of these same inner-development techniques, that you'll spontaneously enter into a full-blown past-life memory experience from time to time, or at least have the total sensation of doing so. In fact, you will enjoy all kinds of visions and revelations concerning what happens after you cross that final frontier. But as the Zen master said to the student who came to him exclaiming excitedly about the high quality celestial visions he'd been experiencing, 'Just keep breathing and they'll pass.'

Because what good are these visions to you in this present moment, no matter how precise or even valid they may be? In this present moment, all you know is that you're here. You don't know how long for, but for now you're here.

Surely the truly enlightened approach, the truly Taoist approach, is to adopt a compassionately nihilistic attitude to death and, if you can handle that with aplomb, you'll be well ahead of the game when you actually do drop your body and find that all the time you spent developing immortal spirit body awareness in the fifth dimension was well invested. But the fact is, you won't know till it happens, no matter how much I or anyone else fills your head with conjecture, albeit conjecture steeped in an ancient tradition of enlightenment.

In which case, if you truly want self-empowerment in the moment, this one for example, allow yourself the pleasure of accepting the possibility and, as far as we actually can prove, probability, that when your brain dies, your consciousness will evaporate and all there will be is oblivion. Utter oblivion. Imagine it.

You won't feel pain. You won't feel at all. You simply won't be. The time and space you once occupied will cease to be anything more than a black hole.

Can you go there? Just for a moment? I know it's difficult. I know it makes you shudder.

But if you can train yourself to accept that, you can accept anything. If you can look even oblivion in the eye without becoming internally disassembled, you can face anything this particular lifetime can present you with.

If you can accept oblivion, not with false bravado, not in denial of your mortal fear, but in humble acceptance of yourself quaking in your existential boots, you have acquired full warrior status and will notice an amazing surge of energy fill your middle chamber. (That'll be the essence of courage filling you.)

Roll this sentence around in your head: nothing happens when you die.

First entertain it from the above-described nihilistic angle. Then entertain it from the spiritual-romantic angle. For between you and me, no matter how hard I contemplate oblivion, that still small voice inside (that portion of self sequestered in my three inner chambers), whispers, 'No, Doctor, there is no oblivion. Nothing happens when you die! At death you will simply drop your body, that's all. And when you drop your body, you will find yourself where you always were, here in the fifth dimension (for ever and ever).' But don't take too much notice of that, even if it does tally with all Taoist and, to some extent, Buddhist and Hindu so-called data on the subject.

Even if it tallies with what you instinctively know, take it with a pinch of salt.

Because, as I said, no one alive, not now, or in the past, no matter how venerable or learned, knows doodly squat when it comes to death.

Even though it's comforting to think otherwise. But then comfort never made for a proper adventure. And as a proper adventure is what you're on and not a dress rehearsal, it would be wise (if you want to maintain a modicum of honesty with yourself) to embrace the insecurity of not having a clue what happens after you die and prepare yourself for absolute oblivion, just in case you get disappointed (not that you'd know).

You may think I am pussyfooting here (as opposed to barefooting), but that's because I truly can't bring myself to say anything that could fill you with false hope. I can only tell you what my inner self believes, or thinks it believes, in the light of thirty years' meditation practice (as described in this book), which is that it's perfectly OK to believe your consciousness will go on for ever like this, as long as you don't take your beliefs seriously.

The point is, whether you subscribe to the nihilistic Taoist view of oblivion or the spiritual- romantic Taoist view of golden immortals riding the backs of the seven celestial winds, you're here now, so it doesn't really matter. There'll be plenty of time to deal with whatever occurs or doesn't when you get there (or don't).

In essence, both the nihilistic and eternalistic approaches are just that – approaches. Try suspending judgement and not buying into either so you remain in the innocent 'what next?' state as much of the time as possible.

To help you adopt this enlightened, devil-may-care Taoist attitude to your own (upcoming) demise, and thus further develop courage in day-to-day or night-to-night matters (out on the street), lie, sit or stand comfortably. Ensure maximum mainframe expansion, muscles at full sinking and relaxation, optimum fluidity, evenness and depth of breathing, and situate yourself in triplicate in your trio of inner chambers, witnessing from the upper, feeling from the middle and driving from the lower.

While maintaining such inner assemblage, become aware of your own skeleton – to the exclusion of all other mainframe aspects. You are simply your skeleton. You are now simply a collection of bones – skull bones (66 in all), spinal vertebrae, clavicle (collarbone), sternum (breastbone), ribs, scapulae (shoulder blades), upper arm bones, forearm bones, hand bones, finger bones, pelvic bones, pubic bone, thigh bones, lower leg bones, foot bones and toe bones.

As you breathe in, feel the subtle breath permeate you as this collection of bones imbuing them (you) with strength and, as you breathe out, feel the subtle breath flow throughout the skeleton body and all brittleness leave you. Maintain this until you rather enjoy just being a skeleton.

Now extend awareness to all the soft tissue in your body—muscles, tendons, ligaments, fascia (connective tissue), organ tissue, blood vessel tissue, gland tissue, nerve tissue, brain tissue and so on – and be nothing but the skeleton body and tissue body.

As you inhale, let subtle breath permeate your tissue body as well as your skeleton body. As you exhale, let the subtle breath extend to all parts of your tissue and skeleton bodies and all weariness leave you. Remain like this, breathing in and out until you feel comfortable as just flesh and bones.

Now let awareness extend to all the fluids in your body – blood, cerebrospinal fluid, synovial fluid (in the joints), lymph, digestive juices, sweat, tears, mucous, urine and so on – and simply be the fluid body (as well as the skeleton body and tissue body).

As you inhale, let subtle breath permeate all the fluid body as well as the tissue body and skeleton body. As you exhale, let the subtle breath radiate to all parts and all stagnation leave you. Remain like this, breathing in and out until you're happy just being fluid, tissue and bones.

Now extend awareness to all the nerves in your body, both the sympathetic system and parasympathetic, and simply be the nerve body (as well as the fluid, tissue and skeleton bodies).

As you inhale, let subtle breath permeate your nerves as well as your fluids, tissue and bones.

As you exhale, let subtle breath radiate to all parts and all confusion leaves you. Remain like this breathing in and out until it feels quite natural to be just the nerves, fluids, tissue and bones.

Now let awareness extend to your internal meta-network of energy super-conduits and general network of organ and bowel related meridians – your energy body, in other words –and simply be your energy body (as well as your nerve body, fluid body, tissue body and skeleton body).

As you inhale, let subtle breath permeate your energy body, as well as your nerve, fluid, tissue and skeleton bodies.

As you exhale, let subtle breath radiate to all parts and all inertia leave you. Remain like this breathing in and out until it feels satisfying to be merely the energy, nerves, fluid, tissue and bones.

Now extend awareness to your spirit body (from the three inner chambers out to the edges of your protective energy shield) and simply be the spirit body (as well as the energy, nerve, fluid, tissue and skeleton bodies).

As you inhale, let subtle breath permeate your spirit body, as well as your energy, nerve, fluid, tissue and skeleton bodies.

As you exhale, let subtle breath radiate to all parts and all ignorance leave you. Remain like this breathing in and out, simply being your spirit, energy, nerves, fluid, tissue and bones until it feels quite ordinary just being that.

You may notice at this point or some time later that the only thing that makes you recognize that collection of bodies as 'you' is your mind, and more specifically various intricately interwoven complexes of habitual thought patterns in 'your' mind that keep reaffirming, This is me!'

Instead, at each stage of the above meditation, you could affirm, 'This is not me,' that is if you're serious about all this enlightenment business.

The effect of this is to help you gradually disidentify from the body in order to dissipate fear of the body's eventual demise, while at the same time enabling you to feel more comfortable taking it up as your temporary residence or vehicle while you're still fortunate enough to 'have' it (large). Talking of which, if you wish to extend that tenancy as far as you possibly can into the future, you may like to indulge in some light-hearted banter with the following group of little treasures. However, if self-destructiveness is getting the better of you and you'd rather hurry up and get it all over with, leave these well alone.

GROUP OF LITTLE TREASURES

If you want to extend life span potential and expand moment-to-moment somatic pleasure and energy response levels, thus augmenting the spirit-body development process, try the following. While sitting or standing, adjust mainframe for maximum vertical and horizontal expansion, muscles for full relaxation and 'sunkenness', especially your neck, shoulders and arms, and breathing for optimum fluidity, evenness and depth. Assemble yourself internally in your trio of inner chambers, observing from the upper, feeling from the middle and driving from the lower, at least for the duration of the following experiment (or evermore if you can manage it). Make loose fists in both hands and using your knuckles, percuss lightly with fast, even tempo and velocity, all over your skull.

Make sure you cover all parts of the cranium as you perform a dexterous, rhythmical drum roll (with shoulders, arms, elbows and wrists completely loose and relaxed), including your forehead, but especially the back of your head on the occipital bone. This is traditionally known as 'beating the heavenly drum', and is highly effective for waking up your brain and stimulating awareness in your upper chamber, as well as promoting blood flow to the scalp to help prevent balding and improve the luster of your hair. A minute or two will suffice to adequately stimulate circulation to all parts of the cranium.

Now, using the little finger edges of your fists, percuss likewise on your chest, beginning in the middle of the breastbone and gradually working your way bilaterally, diagonally upwards along your pectoral muscles towards your shoulders.

As well as releasing tension from the chest and stimulating circulation in the lung and heart region to help support your cardiovascular and respiratory systems, this will stimulate awareness in your middle chamber. It will also help to clear away emotional blockages and make your voice sound more resonant and mellifluous. A minute or two is enough.

Now draw your arms back behind you and using the backs of your fists, percuss the kidney area of your lower back either side of your spine just below your bottom rear ribs and just above the line of your hip bones.

As well as helping to relieve muscular strain in the lumbar region, improve circulation to the kidneys and, by extension, strengthen the entire system, this will stimulate awareness in your lower chamber and increase libido levels. Perhaps not as much as taking Viagra, watching a blue movie or shagging someone you've been lusting after cravenly, but it will make a noticeable difference in the longer term if practiced daily. A minute or two is enough unless feeling particularly frigid, impotent or aching backed, in which case percuss for up to five minutes (if you can).

After percussing all three regions, corresponding to your three inner chambers, lie, sit or stand for a moment or two, appropriately internally assembled and enjoy the after-vibrations as they reverberate throughout your internal somatic architecture. But before this treatise starts to verge on the mundane (earthly or physical in other words), I hope you won't mind if we turn everything on its head.

TURNING THE WORLD ON ITS HEAD

Maintaining the clarity necessary to negotiate your way smoothly through the apparent ups and downs of daily or nightly life, requires a certain agility and flexibility of perspective.

As previously explained, all reality is subjective and therefore relative to your viewing position. Paradoxically, the more easily and instantly you can shift your viewing position in relation to what's going on around you, the more constant and stable will be your inner assemblage and the less your feathers will be ruffled by those (perceived) ups and downs.

Moreover, what you take as given empirical fact is often nothing more than collective delusion. Perceived external conditions that appear to shape your world and define (and limit) your choices are often no more substantial than deft conjuring tricks.

The fundamental basis of four-dimensional reality, in which your local consciousness enjoys its globally urbanized existence, is often ignored or distorted in order to uphold certain cultural myths embedded deep in the collective psyche. Substituting the fundamentals with myth holds you in thrall to potentially unhealthy group delusion, reduces your range of vision and limits your range of response to whatever crops up along your path. Obviously the wider your range of possible responses to whatever crops up, the more chance you have to manage yourself successfully and the less likely you are to become internally disassembled.

And as the integrity of your internal assemblage is crucial to maintaining a modicum of continuous sanity in such turbulent times, it will benefit you to divest yourself immediately of one of the most basic delusions commonly subscribed to and hitherto held sacrosanct.

Dating back to the time people assumed the Earth to be flat and something you'd fall off the edge of if you strayed too far, is a belief, unchallenged by our having discovered the planet's innate roundness, that the sky is 'up' and the ground 'down'. Hence an elevator climbs 'up' to the top of a skyscraper and goes back 'down' to the lobby (or basement if you need to get your car from the underground car park, for example).

But if you're actually on a round planet in infinite space, it is patently absurd to think of 'up' and 'down' as anything more than relative descriptions. More accurate would be to say, 'in' and 'out', where 'in' refers to the Earth's core and 'out' refers to the surrounding atmosphere and space beyond.

To examine the validity of this, orient yourself briefly. Face eastwards in the direction of both the Earth's axial rotation and its heliocentric orbit, and see yourself 'planted' on this round globe, with the soles of your feet pointing in towards the Earth's core and your head pointing out into the atmosphere. From this perspective it soon becomes apparent that even our most cherished concepts of daily life, sunrise and sunset, the daily beginning and end of life-giving light and warmth, are utterly invalid. The sun obviously does not rise in the east, nor set in the west. This is merely an illusion, a trick of the light caused by the still collectively embedded belief in a static flat Earth. In fact, as every schoolchild knows, relative to the Earth, the sun remains still, and it is the Earth rotating in an easterly direction towards the light of the sun that makes the sun look like it's rising in the east. As that rotation continues (at a more or less steady 1,000 miles per hour) through the day, it then appears some hours later that the sun is setting in the west. In fact, that's just an illusion caused by the Earth, or that spot of Earth upon which you're currently situated, rotating away from the sun's light.

So there's no sunrise or sunset in physical four-dimensional reality then, just the axial rotation of the Earth's axis, as it orbits the sun (at this very moment, not in some theoretical realm of science or fantasy) at a staggering 66,000 miles per hour.

There's nothing very static about it either. It just appears nice and still when you're on it because speed is relative and to appreciate it you'd have to be standing on a platform far out in space.

This in no way, however, diminishes the awesome reality that you (and I) are currently hurtling through the depths of infinite space at 66,000 miles per hour (19 miles per second) on the surface of a planet rotating on its axis at 1,000 miles per hour. Remembering and tuning into this is reassuring when local events seem too fast to handle –the high speed of post-modern life is mere child's play by comparison. Such conscious self-orientation also helps you regain perspective when local events seem too big to handle. For compared to such scale, local events assume their proper (minuscule) proportion.

Any time you feel wobbled by local events and are in danger of losing perspective, reorient yourself literally, like this, by facing east (the Orient) and allowing yourself the conscious experience of riding a planet through space at such breakneck speed as this. (You don't have to imagine it, because it's actually happening to you now – simply internally assemble yourself in your three inner chambers and experience it from there.)

However, all this flexing and bending of perspective can be initially tricky on account of how deeply the flat-static-Earth, up-down, day-night myth is embedded in the collective psyche.

For this reason, the cyclically minded Taoists developed a dastardly method of internally turning the world upside down and though sometimes this can cause queasiness if practiced to extreme, it will have an immediately enlightening effect on your current perspective.

Sitting or standing, attend to all rudimentary mainframe adjustment preliminaries, breathe and internally assemble yourself in triplicate in your trio of inner chambers, witnessing from the upper, feeling from the middle and driving from the lower.

Now simply reverse the up-down spatial poles so that the ground is 'up' and the sky is 'down'. You are now as a bat hanging down off the floor, your head pointing down to the ceiling. Now the skyscraper's elevator leaves lobby level and travels down the shaft to the tip (no longer top) of the building, which now represents the lowest point you can reach before actually falling down through the sky.

Look down at the ceiling, then look up at the floor. Keep doing this until you feel just as comfortable as you normally do when the illusion is reversed as previously described.

This encourages a deeper appreciation of the value of the Earth's gravitational force, without which you'd fall immediately down onto the ceiling, probably causing enough damage to require a replastering job. It also gives you enough flexibility of perspective to be able to manage yourself with the minimum of internal dishevelment when the external conditions of your life conspire to turn your world upside down. 'Upside down?' you'll think, 'I can do upside down!'

Talking of which nothing (much) is so capable of turning your world upside down and testing your internal assemblage as conducting yourself in the following:

ONGOING, INTIMATE, ONE-TO-ONE, ROMANTICALLY OR SEXUALLY BASED RELATIONSHIPS

There is nothing much more beautiful than the expression of deep love between two people immersed in one of the above. Nothing sweeter than falling asleep in your lover's arms or similarly waking up (ideally without a stiff neck or frozen shoulder). There is nothing more nurturing than that tenderness. Nothing more comforting than basking in that warmth. Even spending interminable hours together watching mind-numbing TV and scoffing Chinese takeaway isn't so bad.

On a good day.

The problem is, as you have no doubt discovered, good days are not the only kind of day. All relationships must, by the immutable law of yin and yang and what goes up must come down, transit through difficult, painful phases in cyclic alternation with easy, pleasurable ones.

And it is during these down phases that you pay the price for all that comfort.

Because you've grown attached, not just to the idea of that person as a font of warm and tender love, not just to the routine of daily and nightly mutual interactions, but to their on-tap energy at your disposal.

And no matter how much you remember to source your energy from within, you will have been lulled during the good times into the dangerous addictive tendency of sucking energy from them (as well as the addiction to them sucking it from you).

Indeed, one-to-one, intimate, romantically or sexually based relationships offer the richest seam of externally siphoned energy in existence. No amount of money, possessions, achievements, status or temporal power can offer more.

So when this energy is denied you, whether through temporary or permanent breakdown of communication and mutual trust, your (internal) world is thrown upside down causing potentially monumental internal, and often external, dishevelment.

This happens because comfort induces laziness. Laziness induces forgetfulness. And forgetfulness induces you to forget that your energy is best sourced within. Forgetting this causes confusion on an existential level. In that confusion you realize you mistook the relationship as your primary relationship and lost yourself in it, when all along your primary relationship was, in fact, the one you've been conducting with your own self since the day you were conceived and probably will be long after you die. The external relationship with your lover, was in fact your secondary relationship all along. Not that it appears that way during the up-phase. Far from it.

Which is not in any way to recommend avoiding getting involved with people, or staying involved. After all, why make life easy if you can make it difficult?

And during down-phases, relationships are nothing if not difficult. Painfully difficult sometimes. But I don't need to tell you that.

Which is why it's so important not to waste these inevitable down-phases in a relationship or intervals between relationships, as opportunities to reacquaint yourself with the object of your true primary relationship – yourself. Or more specifically that aspect of self that coexists with your local self, interdimensionally and specifically within your three inner chambers.

Because the more strongly identified you are with that font of energy within, the less you'll be lulled into forgetfulness and ensuing energy leeching during the up-phase (or new external relationship) that will inevitably follow (if you want it to).

As well as making you more self-contained, self-sufficient and energy-efficient over the long term, maintaining an ongoing mindful and awake relationship with yourself will expand your capacity to express love more freely and to receive it likewise, while reducing your dependency tendency.

In other words, don't look to others, however close they may (appear) to be to you, for your salvation. Instead, return to yourself, where one internal assemblage has been adequately re-established, you will find salvation in bucketfuls. Not that you actually need saving – you just may think you do – a moment's self-identification with your own immortal spirit body via all aforementioned means will confirm that for you – you don't have to take my word for it.

Relationships revolving around mutual energy leeching – co-dependent ones in other words – involve power and control as their currency. Relationships involving two energy self-sourcing parties, each sharing the fruits of that energy self-sourcing and thus producing synergy, have freedom as their currency, which is after all what any urban warrior values most highly.

So, in practice, when in the doldrums and internally disheveled over a down-phase in your relationship with a 'love-partner', or a complete break with that partner, focus your valuable attention on re-establishing your primary internal relationship with yourself. Once balance is retrieved, your external relationship will then automatically reflect that balance and harmony will prevail again.

This applies as much whether you stay with the external relationship you're 'in', or run away to find another (victim). Whether you want to get in, stay in or get out, always focus your attentions primarily on your own inner balance according to all previously detailed instructions, and outer balance will occur of itself.

Which is all relatively easy to say, but in practice self-retrieval after a good upside-downing tends to be a rather tumultuous process, often giving rise to great inner turbulence before sanity is restored. Sometimes it just makes you want to run (away). Those Taoists of old knew of this escapist tendency and learned to harness its energy for more self-creative purposes in the following manner.

FLYING ON LAND

Picture yourself now, with mainframe at full expansion, breathing regulated and awareness appropriately internally assembled to facilitate full spirit-body identification, running effortlessly away from all your troubles. Imagine that with every step you take, you (as spirit body) are propelled huge distances at inconceivable speed. Imagine this to be so much the case that you could, if you wished, hop from planet to planet and work your way round the entire universe within a matter of hours and be home in time for lea, hardly breathless and with not a drop of perspiration to be seen.

If your imagination won't stretch to such universal proportions, imagine yourself completing a three-mile course in seconds.

If you have the interest you can develop this internal technique to use as a method of astral projection, by taking advantage of the previously described etheric web, for purposes of distant healing or message delivery when your mobile battery's dead or your server's broken down.

Alternatively, you can use it as inner template and actually take your mainframe out on the street for a walk or a run and give your immortal spirit body a good airing.

Such activity was traditionally known as 'flying on land' and many legends arose of practitioners who could walk or run two or three hundred miles in a day without fatigue. Though this was probably a case of exaggeration by Chinese whisper, it nevertheless remains true that flying on land is a great way to get around.

Walking or running, according to your inclination, (with eyes open) maintain awareness in your three inner chambers, witnessing from the upper, feeling from the middle and driving your mainframe movement from the lower. Let yourself shed all sense of local identity progressively more with each successive step so that, in no time at all, you feel yourself to be nothing more than any old mainframe and spirit body moving along the street (or wherever). In other words, drop the weight of your life story to date from your shoulders.

Let your shoulders relax completely. Let your whole body relax completely and breathe in time with your footsteps by inserting a slight pause halfway through the inhalation and another halfway through the exhalation. By this I mean breathe in, pause, breathe in more, breathe out, pause, breathe out more, breathe in, and so on. Coincide the first part of the inhalation with one step, the second part with the next, the first part of the exhalation with the next step and the last part with the next, and so on.

This form of control, known traditionally as 'four-stage breathing' prevents your heart from overloading and stops you getting out of breath, no matter what distance you cover.

At all times ensure your spine is fully lengthened to prevent compression at the back of your neck and keep your footsteps light as if trying not to disturb the Earth's vibrations any more than they already are. This is so as not to jar your joints or cause undue muscular tension, especially in the shoulder and upper back region, which is susceptible to misalignment leading to spinal problems, especially from running.

The idea is for the mainframe to be so aligned and relaxed that you're hardly aware of it, leaving you free to experience the motion of walking or running or even skipping along if you wish (fantastic down hill and mountain sides), as pure spirit.

To help you achieve this weightless 'cheetah' state, turn the world upside down as before (to take the weight off your feet) and imagine yourself to be walking on the spot – as if on a treadmill pedaling the ground beneath your feet in the manner of a performing seal pedaling a (very large) ball.

Additionally, visualize a strand of etheric fiber, composed, if the fancy takes you, of ultra-bright electric blue light (etheric substance), extending from your lower chamber to your intended (external) destination and imagine it pulling you effortlessly towards that point as if by exportation.

If walking, allow your arms to swing naturally from the shoulder joints, with palms turned slightly towards to scoop up chi from the air. If running, bend your arms at the elbows and turn your palms upwards at waist height as if carrying your invisible golden morphing energy ball.

See all the scenery passing you by – including people, animals, birds, fish, insects, reptiles, billboards, traffic lights, buildings, cars, boats, trains, planes, trees, shrubbery, vast tracts of industrial wasteland, pleasant green fields, oceans, mountains, mobile-phone transmission masts and anything else you can think of – as manifestations of the Tao, that invisible natural force that generates and informs the existence of all that is.

As you walk or run along, keep (silently) saying to the Tao, take my troubles away from me! Take my troubles away from me! Take my troubles away from me!'

Don't make a big deal out of flying on land. No special time is required to practice it. Simply include it as part of your routine transportation program, perhaps taking advantage of your journeys to work and back to walk or run part of the way in flying mode.

You can of course apply this technique of using correct mainframe awareness, relaxation, four-stage breathing and proper spirit body awareness enhancing self-assemblage in your inner chambers, as well as turning the world upside down and extending the blue light from your lower chamber, to all forms of exercise no matter what. Your movement, whether in the process of dancing, weight-training, rock climbing, snowboarding, cycling, circuit training, yoga or martial arts, for instance, will be intelligent movement, as opposed to the goal-orientated, bulging-templed, huffing-and-puffing and, it must be said, highly idiotic movement we are more familiar with in post-modern Western society.

However, sometimes the stress of efficiently handling all the details in a busy urban day or night will overcome you, no matter how intelligently you move through your agenda, which as you know can contribute to an accumulation of irritability, frustration or downright rage. To prevent you succumbing unwisely to possible urges to express this violently, either towards self in the form of self-destructive habit indulgence or towards others as unwarrior-like violent or aggressive behavior you'd later have cause to regret, those old Taoists (who though they lived in the ancient Orient were no strangers to things that can piss you off during a busy day or night) developed the following methods of safe but effective anger release.

SAFE BUT EFFECTIVE ANGER RELEASE FOR URBAN WARRIORS

Unless you are a dictator of a well-armed country with the military in your pocket or just a plain thug, it is always wiser not to vent your frustrations through hostile, aggressive or violent behavior towards others. You can, of course, use your anger as part of a strategy to protect human life (yours or someone you're protecting) in the face of imminent physical attack – when not sufficiently trained in the art of self-defense to fight without anger.

Even if you appear to come out on top of the situation in the short term, you will, if possessed of only a modicum of sensibility, be filled with a growing sense of shame for acting like such a beast of the field; a sense of shame you will find hard to reconcile with the finer warrior qualities you possess. This will mean many wasted minutes on the phone to friends in a bid for assurance that you're not such a dickhead as your outburst led you to believe you were, and all to no avail, because in that instance you were a dickhead. Not that there's anything so terrible about being a dickhead (I'm often one myself), just as long as it doesn't become habitual.

We all make mistakes. It's an inevitable part of the ride down the great thoroughfare, but it's obviously something you would wish, as a warrior, to keep to a minimum – especially in connection with the inappropriate expression of rage, if only to save valuable time spent in subsequent damage limitation exercises, custodial sentences or hospital.

To this end, if you want to communicate your anger effectively to someone (who has roused your ire), expand your mainframe, breathe, relax and say (aloud – to them), 'I feel angry because it seems to me you're doing such and such and I'd rather you did such and such.' Obviously you can expand the such and such sections to include all relevant data. And if addressing someone far larger, stronger, bestial, more well-armed or wearing navy blue, black or camouflage outfit bearing the word 'police' or 'military', or indeed someone with the power to wreck your career, substitute the word 'angry' for 'upset'.

That's basic communication skills, but to release a charge of stored rage held for someone in particular, where the sensible expression of that rage would be inappropriate, sit or stand with feet 2 feet apart, knees bent, mainframe at maximum expansion, muscles relaxed and sunk, breathing regulated, awareness properly situated in your three inner chambers and slowly turn your waist from side to side. As you do so, let this motion naturally allow your arms to alternately fly out softly in front of you at chest height with palms open until each arm reaches almost to full extension, pulling the fingers back at the last second to form a fist. In other words, throw punches, one arm after the other, only forming fists when the arm is almost at full stretch to produce a whipping action similar to flicking your school tie (if you're old enough to remember such things) in someone's face.

Visualize the person to whom your anger is directed standing before you in such a way as to receive these punches fully in the face. As you punch away at them, repeat in time with each punch, 'I hate you, I hate you, I hate you!' After a few minutes of this, start reminding yourself that that person is actually doing the very best they can according to their current stage of personal evolution and that there is no need for you to take the effects of that personally. Once remembered, start saying, 'I love you, I love you, I love you!' until you get a moment's sense of what the words mean, then stop punching them. After all, why beat the shit out of someone.

For a more immediate release of generalized frustration, or even just to clear your head, sit or stand, internally accommodated as before.

Inhale. As you do so, make fists and gather your arms into a circle on the horizontal plane at chest height as if holding a fat vertical roll of carpet to your chest, with fists pressed firmly together at the knuckles. For a moment, contrary to the general rule of never holding your breath before exhaling, hold your breath, while imagining all your frustration compressed into the space in front of your chest (formerly) occupied by the imaginary carpet roll.

Count to three and on three fling your arms open, releasing your fists, into the wide open embrace position, while allowing to escape from the depths of your belly, out through your open throat and mouth, the very loud, very sudden, very powerful sound, 'HAAAAAAH!!!!' until all your breath is exhaled. As the sound escapes, see the ball of former frustration leave you and roll off like a thunderbolt into the great beyond to be transformed into something more useful.

Drop your arms slowly to your sides and spend an empty moment in the silence of the aftershock.

Be sure to keep your throat open and relaxed while the sound is escaping to avoid becoming hoarse.

As well as being a powerful frustration release tool, this 'Taoist yell' was also traditionally used to induce terror in one's opponent and to engender courage in the yeller before a fight or in order to prevent one developing. You may find it useful in that respect yourself one day.

It is best to give voice to a good yell like this on some kind of regular basis if you want to allay the inevitable escalation of inner frustration that comes with living in such generally crowded conditions on the planet.

However, this may prove impractical in respect of appropriate yelling space, in which case, while out and about, though preferably in open parkland, it is perfectly permissible to yell for your imaginary dog it you don't have a real one. The dog's name I personally use is 'Rowley', not for any particular reason other than it's an easy sound to yell without straining my vocal cords. When doing so, you need entertain no fears about being thought deranged, as long as you act as if you are actually calling for your dog who seems to have run off far into the distance. So no self-consciousness after the yell, just carry on walking and act natural, enjoying the release of energy and ready to face whatever is coming next.

FACING WHATEVER IS COMING NEXT

Your face is literally (he point of interface between you and the external world. Other than your hairstyle, general mainframe shape and the apparel you drape upon and about it, your face is what people recognize you by, visually at least. It is also the part of you through whose agency you literally face the external world as well as all the plans, fears and expectations you harbor about facing it.

As a result, tension easily accrues in your facial musculature, in turn causing a certain tension throughout your cranium. This impedes circulation of blood, cerebrospinal fluid and energy to the brain and upper chamber in particular, rendering you less capable of thinking clearly or positively in relation to whatever it is you're facing up to.

Moreover, your face is the site of a pattern of reflex points relating to your various internal organs much in the same way as the soles of your feet, your palms, your ears and even, would you believe, your external genitalia. Imagine a scaled down human body standing in crucifix posture, with an arm extended over each eyebrow (on your face).Thus the (scaled down) head will be just above the bridge of your nose and the torso suspended over each cheek, its pelvic floor in line with the base of your chin (and its legs hanging down like a strange cravat over your throat).Thus by stimulating with massage, pressure or acupuncture needle, for example, the points three quarters of an inch bilaterally below the corners of your mouth on the fleshy part of your chin, you will simultaneously stimulate your kidneys by reflex.

The Taoists of old discovered that if you were to systematically stretch the muscles of your face (and tongue) on a regular basis, you would stimulate the flow of energy (indirectly by reflex) throughout your entire mainframe, increase circulation throughout the cranium directly and so increase positive clear thinking. You would also increase flexibility of the facial muscles to allow more variation of facial expression, so making you more interesting to watch (on TV or elsewhere), and indirectly, through metaphorical association, this would help you face the world more readily. To top it all, these exercises would also make you look damn good (as does exercise make any body part). Facial exercise was thus quickly adopted by all the vain bastards of the imperial court and became known affectionately as 'those Taoist facial rejuvenation exercises' (except in Mandarin).

Specifically (unless you don't want to lend your features the appearance of someone ten years younger or prefer to be as facially unremarkable as possible), adjust mainframe, breathing and inner assemblage for optimum relaxation and awareness, inhale and gently elongate your face as much as possible, your forehead pulling up towards the lop of your head, your eye sockets opening wide, nostrils flaring, your upper lip stretching down over your gums and your chin stretching down towards your chest. (Hey, why the long face!)

Exhale and scrunch your face up as small as if will go so you look like a mean little mother.

Repeat this slowly up to 18 times, then rest (your face) and enjoy the warmth as the circulation increases.

This both stimulates all the reflex points on your face so benefiting all your internal organs and generally loosens cranial tension thus increasing circulation of blood, energy and cerebrospinal fluid to your brain.

Now, breathing steadily, rotate your chin (and jaw), in the manner of a camel chewing, up to 18 times in each direction with lips slightly apart. Then immediately rotate your tongue tip around the outside of your gums up to 18 times in each direction.

Straightaway gently knock your upper and lower teeth together (very lightly) up to 36 times.

Now rest (your face) and enjoy the sensation of increased circulation around your chin and gums and along the length of your tongue. Not only does this help keep your gums healthy, loosen your jaw tension and stimulate your all-important (in age management terms) pituitary gland (above the roof of your mouth), but it also makes you far more adroit when it comes to kissing and oral sex (obviously).

Breathing fluidly, now raise and lower your entire forehead quite quickly up to 81 times focusing on the muscles around your eyes stretching and relaxing. You will also feel a corresponding movement at the base of your skull. Be sure to do this gently and in a relaxed way.

When you have finished, rest for a moment and enjoy the warmth from the increase of circulation at the back of your skull, through your forehead and around your eyes.

This tones the muscles around your eyes and helps to reduce the ageing effects of bags and lines, helps reduce forehead tension, especially frown lines and the vertical liver-tension lines between your eyebrows, as well as stimulate the optical cortex at the back of your head, helping to strengthen eyesight.

Now, breathing fluidly, with your lips together, pull your chin downwards and inwards towards your throat, so it feels like your jowls (if you had any) are being stretched downwards towards your collar bone, and release. Repeat this quite quickly up to 81 times and relax.

This helps relax and strengthen your jaw and makes your mouth more flexible and so nicer to look at and to kiss (if ever you should find yourself in such a position).

Inhale. As you do so, open your mouth as wide as possible into the biggest (fake) smile you can manage, while attempting to keep the rest of your face, including your eyes, as relaxed as possible.

Exhale and relax. Repeat this slowly up to 18 times and rest, enjoying the pleasure of increased circulation to mouth and jaw.

This basically stretches your smile capacity making you better company (especially at cocktail parties).

Finally, inhale. As you exhale, open your mouth as wide as it will go, extend your tongue as far as it will stretch over your chin and simultaneously open your eyes as wide as possible and look up as if trying to see the crown of your own head. Be careful to look up gently to avoid detaching your retinas.

Repeat this up to 18 times and rest in the luxurious feeling of increased circulation throughout your face, skull and throat.

This will kick-start circulation to your ocular (eyeball) region and stimulate your pituitary gland and, more importantly, your thyroid gland (in your throat). It can also be an effective way to ease a sore throat. I won't even mention the beneficial effects I've heard described by practitioners of the ancient and venerable art of fellatio.

Obviously, regular morning practice of these stretches will quickly improve your appearance. At least that's the hook, because we all want to look good (usually above all else). But the real benefit, apart from greater relaxation and command of facial expression, is the increase in willingness and readiness to face whatever's coming next. Which right now happens to be the following.

CALLING IN THE FOUR GOLDEN IMMORTALS

Moving right along now from the (sur)face of things in a backward flowing direction (still remember that!) to the depths once more, before beginning the slow and gentle re-entry process that'll leave you closing the book ready to launch yourself into a whole new phase of adventure. It's time to call in the Four Golden Immortals – Andy, Quimper, Joel and Lando (kidding, absolutely).

Though the tendency to personify spiritual forces is a childlike device for scaling down concepts too magnitudinous to grasp in any other way, there are times or moods when with all the spiritual sophistication in the world, it simply feels right (and I emphasize the word, 'feels').

Spiritual force, or let's say for the sake of convenience, the Tao, is essentially ineffable (though admittedly I've tried to 'eff' about it a bit in this book). The personification of something entirely unpersonifiable obviously makes no sense to you as a streetwise intelligent being. However, it makes sense to that crucial childlike part of you that resonates with the non-logical, non-rational, mythological, symbolic level of so-called reality. A fantasy reality where a god can descend from the fifth dimension, have sexual intercourse with a human female who lives just a few miles from the eastern shores of the Mediterranean (only a relatively short while before the birth of extensive mass tourism in that region), get her pregnant with a boy who grows up as a carpenter (influence of his mum's side of the family) who becomes an avatar (his dad's influence), gets brutally murdered by the authorities after being grassed up for being a dangerous dissident, rises from the dead, goes off to give his friends a shock, disappears in a cloud and winds up being the biggest celebrity on the planet ever. Even bigger than his mother or any of her subsequent namesakes – and that's big – beyond 'A-list' at least. And it all makes perfect sense.

What I'm saying, excuse the irreverence and thank Christ they don't burn heretics these days, is if you'll swallow that you'll swallow anything, including this Four Golden Immortals story. But do so remembering that no matter how fervently we cherish the idea of Great Grandfather (Wakantanka), the Great Spirit, Jah, Jehova, Brahma, Christ, Krishna, Ganesh (I love you, elephant dude), the Great Mother, Isis, Mary (Our Blessed Lady, blessed be she), Shiva, Buddha, Narayan, Lakshmi (go on girl!), the Great Kahuna, Abraxus, Zoroastra, somebody I'm purposely not mentioning in case of terrorist reprisals, God (of course), Hanuman, or the entire host of angelic and saintly presences belonging to any or all of the above camps, they merely represent inadequate, albeit obviously well-intentioned, sketches of some of the infinite faces of the supreme facelessness, the ineffable, Tao (or whatever goddamn name you want to call it).

I am not espousing atheism, mind you. I wouldn't wish to get involved with your business to that extent. No, this is the exact opposite to atheism. This is pure 'ism'.

That's why (as a pure 'isist', or Taoist, for the sake of phonetic ease) it's perfectly valid and highly advisable to talk to deities you love as if they were huge skybound people whenever you feel the inclination. Praying is one of the most beautiful activities a warrior can engage in. And there is no doubt that all your prayers are heard – though you might not always get the answer you think you want.

There is nothing that will connect the essential child in you to the Tao more than a heart (middle chamber) full of prayer.

But let's not mystify ourselves to the degree of confusion that would have us fight wars over which face of the faceless is better.

Instead, on finding yourself in holy communion with one such divine face of the faceless divine, give yourself in totality to the experience – even say a prayer for me if you want – but remember you are talking to none other than yourself. Not in a deluded schizophrenic way (hopefully), but in the full knowledge (as previously given) that your prayer is received and processed by that part of you that exists for all time in the fifth dimension and which is etherically connected, and so one with, the ineffable, interdimensional, ubiquitous presence, or Tao (aka all the above mentioned).

With that (heresy) in mind, give yourself to the experience of meeting the Four Golden Immortals, who will, from the goodness of their hearts (middle chambers), surround you wherever you go from now on, for the rest of your life and probably beyond, like a quartet of spirit-minders with (etheric) dark suits, shades and trilbies – if you ask them nicely.

Before you think of doing that though, it would be best if you were clued up on what they can do for you.

The 'Four Golden Immortals' are beings who attained the fully immortalized state through the same practices as described in this very book, while still in human form. Since which time they've been riding the backs of the seven winds for aeons, celestially cavorting in carefree abandon and both willing and desirous to share their infinite pleasure with anyone who's interested. This is not because of a desire to do good, it is simply their innate nature to be so. It comes gratis. You owe nothing in return. Though obviously the more you give of the gifts you receive, the more you receive to 'replace' what you've given.

Each of the four has a different set of qualities to pass on to you. And you can take as much as you want. The more you take, the more they give you. Obviously if you don't share of these qualities – if you suppress them and prevent them from inspiring and informing your external actions – they will go to waste.

So the idea is to call in the quartet and refill on a regular enough basis to facilitate a surplus you simply can't help sharing automatically.

In short, these guys (ineffable non-human beings) can turn you into an instant holy man or woman, albeit in the funky urban-warrior style of your choice, capable of emanating such spiritual presence you'll be up there on the 'beyond A-list' with Jesus and all the other (usual) suspects in no time. If you don't want such a degree of personal power, therefore, skip instantly to the next item.

When beckoned, these four, who are nameless and so can be named as you like, each more huge and voluminous than the whole of the eastern sky on a sunny day, ride the celestial winds from wherever they are and instantaneously appear in your immediate etheric vicinity (by virtue of the previously described etheric web), arranging themselves without fuss about your etheric person, or spirit body, in the following formation.

To your right, for as far, wide, high and low as the eye can see, is Golden Immortal 'Andy' (or name of your choice), who carries the gifts of love, compassion, grace, courage, beauty and joy, as well as the power to radiate such qualities, the ability to care for (self and) others, in other words.

To your left, for as far, wide, high and low as the eye can see, is Golden Immortal 'Quimper' (or name of your choice), who carries the gifts of strength, power, honor, integrity, virtue, protection and the ability to use those qualities to lead (oneself) and others.

Behind you, for as far, wide, high and low as the eye can see, is Golden Immortal 'Joel' (or name of your choice), who carries the gifts of health, longevity, material abundance and the abilities to express those qualities through healing and prospering (self and) others.

In front of you, for as far, wide, high and low as the eye can see is Golden Immortal 'Lando' (or name of your choice), who carries the gifts of vision, light, wisdom, knowledge, humor and the ability to express those qualities by teaching and entertaining others.

Though (as with herbal medicine) it takes up to three weeks of daily intake before these qualities build up to a noticeable level in the 'bloodstream', if you show them (the fearsome four) the receipt from this book, you'll be entitled to a preliminary trial session with no obligation to sign up.

In fact, forget the receipt and lying, sitting or standing, adjust your mainframe for optimum vertical and horizontal expansion, your muscles for full relaxation and 'sunkenness', your breathing for maximum fluidity, evenness and depth, and your inner assemblage for balanced distribution in triplicate among your three inner chambers, observing from the upper, feeling from the middle and driving from the lower, thus facilitating a moment of spirit body awareness. Spin the subtle breath around your internal meta-network of energy super conduits as previously described if the mood takes you, and proceed as follows.

Silently call, The Four Golden Immortals' (or address as you see fit), and from your upper chamber see them instantaneously arrange themselves in formation around your person, feeling their presence from your middle chamber and driving the sensation from your lower.

Focus awareness to your right and allow that Golden Immortal to inject you with the gifts of love, compassion, grace, courage, beauty and joy, as well as the power to radiate such qualities, the ability to care for (self and) others. Feel these qualities enter your system one by one, like fine but all-powerful vapors, through the right side of your spirit body and filling it entirely and collecting in your penetrating channel (running up and down the length of the front face of your backbone). Acknowledge receipt somehow, by saying, Thank you!' perhaps.

Focus awareness to your left and allow that Golden Immortal to inject you with the gifts of strength, power, honor, integrity, virtue, protection and the ability to use those qualities to lead (oneself) and others. Feel these qualities enter your system one by one, like fine but all-powerful vapors, through the left side of your spirit body, filling it entirely and collecting in your penetrating channel, and acknowledge receipt as before.

Focus awareness behind you and allow that Golden Immortal to inject you with the gifts of health, longevity, material abundance and the ability to express those qualities through healing and prospering (self and) others. Feel these qualities enter your system one by one, like fine but all-powerful vapors, through the back of your spirit body, filling it entirely and collecting in your penetrating channel, and acknowledge receipt as before.

Focus awareness in front of you and allow that Golden Immortal to inject you with the gifts of vision, light, wisdom, knowledge, humor and the ability to express those qualities by teaching and entertaining others. Feel these qualities enter your system one by one, like fine but all-powerful vapors, through the front of your spirit body and filling it entirely and collecting in your penetrating channel and acknowledge receipt as before.

Finally, to give the experience its appropriate metaphysical context, focus awareness simultaneously above, below and all around you, even as far as to encompass the vastness of the fearsome four. Allow yourself the vision of you (your spirit body) and your four minders within an etheric womb, the infinite proportions of which are greater than the greatest expanse of celestial space imaginable, the owner of which is none other than the greatest celestial mother of them all, the one and only living Tao (or whatever you'd prefer to call 'her', but it does have to be a 'her' as a 'him' would be awkward with a womb, no matter 'his' level of omnimorphabilily. And that's not metaphysical sexism.)

See or rather know yourself now, penetrating channel filled to bursting with enough fine qualities to stimulate the automatic, spontaneous expression of divine splendor for 10 thousand lifetimes, supported for all eternity in (possibly) the most accommodating, nurturing, durable (eternal) life support-system ever described by human hand and keyboard.

Feel the essence of all combined qualities currently contained in your penetrating channel now burst out in all directions and radiate throughout your entire spirit body and beyond, to travel along every fibrous strand of the etheric web in every direction at once, thus sharing the mix with all who are open to receive it. And as you give, so shall you receive exponentially multiplied.

It is perfectly valid to maintain constant low-level awareness of part or all of this vision as you go about your day-to-day, night-to-night business from now on for the rest of your life. It certainly won't cramp your style in any way and will, once habitual, enable you to regard others as similarly situated 'in utero'. Full experience of such vision is equivalent to one Western-style old-school epiphany, which is always good value when you're feeling a bit flat or epiphany-deficient.

Of course it's also perfectly permissible to request a quick top-up of any quality you like. If, for example, trying to think more clearly when hung over or attempting to see the way ahead through an existential fog, just call for Lando (or name of your choice) and he (or she) will be there. (Oh yes, lordy, lordy.)

But what if you're simply in one of those self-absorbed moods and feel, just for the hell of it, like developing your psychic power and boosting your confidence when imagining yourself to be a lone urban warrior standing square in the face of the storm? Is there a high-speed device of which you can avail yourself to effect such a state (in a hurry)?

You bet your perineum there is.

And this is how it happens:

THAT OLD HOOK LOOK

You know what they say: 'There's nothing like a hook look.' Until now, however, you probably neither knew what they meant nor even cared.

But if (like those Taoists of old) you were to draw the fingertips of one hand (either hand will do) together to touch the tip of the thumb of that same hand, thus forming a hook shape with that hand, and proceed to position that hand in such a way as to facilitate the physically relaxed and comfortable spatial alignment of eyeball and hook apex, with relevant arm bent at elbow and wrist, and were furthermore to spend a few moments gazing intently at that apex (comprised of congress of thumb and finger tips), with awareness of the flow of chi between eyeball and that apex, and then issue the appropriate internal command, you would no doubt readily agree with them (that there's nothing like that old hook look).

To put it plainly, sit comfortably, attend to all the usual preliminaries, collect the fingertips of say, your right hand around the tip of your (right) thumb to form the point of a 'hook' and with shoulder, neck and arm fully relaxed, position your hand so that you can gaze at the hook point comfortably for a few moments.

As you gaze, keep your eyes soft and relaxed and blink as often as you like. Become aware of a stream of etheromagnetic force running between that point and your eyes, as if holding your invisible morphing golden ball of energy between hook-point and forehead-central (that point between your eyebrows).

Once awareness of this stream is holding steady (at 186,000 miles per second), issue the following commands (express the following sentiments in other words), feeling their import reverberate accordingly throughout your entire (spirit) body:

'I have clear vision. I have strength. I know what I'm doing. Everyone and everything conspires to help me.'

I should point out that this constitutes the making of a positive affirmation, though it is hoped that by setting such an affirmation within a suitable Taoist context, it can remain without faux new-age connotations; connotations that might otherwise prejudice you in favour of dismissing it as something faddish and hence of little value.

On the contrary, making this affirmation on a daily basis, while simultaneously throwing one of those old hook looks, will over time increase your self-confidence. You'll know exactly what's what, have the strength to endure whatever you must, come what may, trust the moment-to-moment as well as momentous decisions you make and feel the support rather than the hindrance of the world around you.

And that's pure urban warrior. It has nothing to do with new age or old age, it's just an appropriate stance for a warrior to adopt on a daily basis in such a potentially dangerous situation as that presented by living on this particular planet at this particular time.

Throwing a look at your hook for a few moments every day, once a week or on any other regular basis of your choice will gradually increase your powers of telepathy, short-term memory recall, mental focus and concentration ability according to the frequency of practice.

To emphasize the psychic development option, supplement this by pressing firmly with thumb, finger, pen-top or any other improvised self-kneading instrument, for a minute or so on those points in the natural depressions formed where the tips of your deltoid (shoulder cap) muscles meet the biceps in your upper arms. These points (officially known by acupuncturists rather unromantically as 'Large Intestine 14') were used in lieu of the internet and mobile telephones by the Taoists of old to maintain 'second sight', 'sixth sense', enhanced extra-sensory perception, or however you'd prefer to think of it, as an adjunct to looking at their hooks.

Try this for a moment or two now and you won't even have to read what's coming next - you'll already know.

But just in case you haven't time ...

TIME AND THE EASY, EFFECTIVE MANAGEMENT THEREOF

As originally stated, there's no time.

The idea of a procession of moments (or temporal units of uniform value forming a continuous strand of linear time) is merely a device we have collectively developed and subscribed to as an unquestionable constant, by which our experience of living on the planet in a physical mainframe can be measured. That's all it is: an idea.

Time, as we generally think of it, is not a constant. Time is, as any Taoist or Einstein will tell you, purely relative. If you're engrossed in the moment, the moment will pass in no time, literally. If you're held internally inert in the grip of self-limiting disengagement – bored, in other words – that moment can last for hours, or at least seem to.

The deeper function of this device we call 'time' is, in fact, to prevent all the events of your life appearing as if they're all happening at once.

For when seen through the eyes of your spirit body – that is, when your spirit body is fully merged in the Tao in the previously described ways, long enough to afford you the clarity to take a glimpse at your life from the (lateral field) perspective of eternity – all the events that comprise your life do in fact all happen at once.

Obviously these are only words, and my using them is not intended to convince you of this, but merely to point out what only becomes obvious when you've seen it. As when finally able to see the hidden 3-D picture (in those hidden 3-D picture things).

But what is immediately apparent, no matter how you look at the picture, is that if duration of time is relative to your quality of experience, it is also susceptible to being stretched or shrunk according to your will – it being none other than you, yourself, who determines or wills your quality of experience with your own mind. Not only is duration susceptible to expansion or contraction, but also to tone control.

You can fill a time span with pleasure or you can fill it with pain according to how you turn the dial.

This will determine the dynamics of your relationship with that time span and dictate whether you view it as friend or foe.

The relevance of this to you as an urban warrior in post-modern, globally urbanized, high-speed life, where there usually appears to be a scarcity of available time spans in which to take care of business adequately at work, rest and play, is to be willing to treat time as your friend. It'll play ball with you and enable you to accomplish everything you want and more. If, on the other hand, you treat time as your enemy, it will become so, and deprive you of valuable moments so you always end up missing deadlines and being late for everything.

Be willing to view the projected time span before you as expansive and able to accommodate all the events with which you desire to fill it, and it will, by the immutable law of yin and yang, the external reflecting the internal and vice versa, bend over backwards to make that possible for you, so friendly is it.

However, view this time span as mean and inadequate, and sure as cosmic egg timers is cosmic egg timers, it will shrink before your very eyes until it disappears into a black hole, and you've missed the moment and its opportunities have passed.

In other words, don't be rude about time, cussing it and exclaiming there isn't enough of the goddamn stuff, and it won't be rude to you.

Conversely, be kind to time and be willing to see its endless possibilities and it'll be kind in return.

But that's the point. When, as an urban warrior, you return to the source of all life within where existence is a constant (eternally), you will trigger the manifestation of endless possibilities within any projected time span, opportunities that otherwise may have lain dormant. That's how the Tao of time works.

And obviously, the more opportunities you have, the greater possibility there is of fulfilling your limitless potential for maximum enjoyment of your life from now on and, by extension, the enjoyment of all those with whom you interact, if only by contagion.

This understanding and appreciation of the malleability of any given time span coupled with a keen ability to prioritize the various projected elements of your intended agenda, as well as a willingness to maintain an appointment book (electronic or paper) and to cross-reference by regularly consulting a reliable timepiece, forms the basis of effective time-management.

But without the following (the other 'D' word), neither time nor indeed any other resource will do you much good. Because you'll be a mess.

DISCIPLINE

Does the very sound of it make you shudder! As any warrior, post-modern or ancient, will tell you, discipline is essential to survival. Not discipline in an obsessive way. Obsession, literally laying siege to someone or thing, removes the object of obsession's breathing space. When someone or something can't breathe, death quickly ensues. And death is the opposite of what we're trying to achieve here.

So no obsession with discipline, simply a willingness to obey your own commands, for to rebel against your own self is patently absurd. Not that that stops us. We all rebel against ourselves to some degree from time to time, doing things we enjoy but which destroy us, peopling this planet the way we do being a case in point, but after all we're human, not machines however hard we try to be otherwise. But as I say, it is a matter of degrees.

Discipline means being willing to obey your own commands enough of the time, without kicking up a fuss, to successfully negotiate your way through any given series of events during any given time span. If you are disciplined you will do this according to the prior parameters and conditions you've determined by conscious choice, without hating yourself for it and so punishing yourself in some underhanded way by preventing yourself from manifesting the outcome you want – which is (I assume) the absolute, unqualified enjoyment of every remaining moment here. (Otherwise, what's the point?)

In other words, there's no point obeying yourself so strictly that you're no longer having fun doing it – if you'll excuse me for mentioning something so trite as fun. But without fun in the moment, without each and every available time span being like a funfair ride, no matter how conditions conspire to make you see otherwise, that time span will drag and thus be a waste (of time).

So really discipline is what enables you to have fun. Discipline, for example, enables you to obey yourself to perform your daily ablutions, without which most polite post-modern society would marginalize you, especially on the cocktail party circuit, and you'd end up all alone and smelly. And that's rarely much fun.

You could in fact make the obvious link and simply say discipline is fun.

Because it's actually fun to command yourself to breathe fluidly, evenly and deeply at this precise moment, for example, and then to experience your body obeying that command and the subsequent sensation of relaxed wellbeing that should hit you just about... now.

It's fun to command your etheric self to resonate with the essence of personal magnetism and then to experience yourself obeying that command only to find beautiful people flocking to you to share the joys of life.

It's fun to command yourself through all the various stages of spirit-body development (as described in this book), to experience the deepest part of you obey those commands and the subsequent profound transformation of both internal and external conditions that will occur.

It's fun to discipline yourself to remember. And it's fun when you forget.

To do otherwise is not the way of the urban warrior, but of the urban degenerate. And though that may get you invited to certain parties where certain twisted people (and the tabloid press if you're infamous enough) can enjoy watching and documenting your self-destruction, degeneration quickly leads to death. A death of which you will not be adequately internally prepared to take full spiritual advantage in the moment. Which would ultimately be a waste as it only happens once (during this particular lifetime at least).

But as I said, it's by degrees. You mustn't be rigid about it. You mustn't be rigid about anything if you want to retain the flexibility of mind and body necessary to roll with the yin and yang of things as they happen and not get caught in an existential slipstream.

Be gentle with yourself. Gentle, but as the old cliché has it, firm. Be the benign dictator who martial led the many selves and made them as one, the wise and compassionate teacher dealing with a child you love – you.

Just don't mistake compassion for indulgence. Though naturally indulgence is inevitable, it is essential you exercise discipline in the areas of self-regeneration such as those described herein, and any others of your choice, in order to offset the degenerative effects of that indulgence.

But always do so in a patient and forgiving way. Self-discipline in no way implies self-flagellation. And talking of self-indulgence ...

WHAT HAPPENS IF YOU MIX THE PILL OF IMMORTALITY WITH OTHER MIND-ALTERING SUBSTANCES!

Whatever you want to happen. That's the way reality works, mind-altering cocktails or not.

Some traditional spiritual systems dictate that the ingestion of any mind-altering substance is counter-productive to self-realization and provides a hindrance to enjoying direct experience of the divine realms. Others insist on the sacramental use of various psychotropic substances on a regular basis in order to enjoy experience of the divine.

On a more mundane level, people have been getting out of their minds using one substance or another since the medicine men (or women) of the wandering clans first started necking the magic mushrooms and offering their urine as free refreshment to the other clan members. Obviously things progressed from that earthy state, till you had us drinking ale from our own mugs and now being able to lay hands (at the drop of a hat) on acid, pills, coke, heroin, ketamine, speed, mushrooms, cannabis, absinthe, tequila or whatever, and doing so en masse, all over the world, every day or night of the week but especially Fridays and Saturdays in unimaginably large (and definitely at least quadruple the amount official figures would have us believe) numbers.

Obviously, I'm not condoning it nor for that matter criticizing it. It's none of my business. What you ingest is entirely your business, as far as I'm concerned. Of course there's a price to pay (as well as the cash). We all know that. But it's your call entirely. Who am I to judge (one way or another)?

Not, I repeat, that I agree with the ingestion of mind-altering substances. Or disagree. It's just a fact of post-modern life that we continue to be in denial about at our peril. So get sharp.

In which light, it is usually recommended that you should not meditate nor engage in any inner-developmental or spiritual exercise while also under the influence of (other) mind-altering substances.

However, as it is unrealistic to expect anyone for whom drugs or alcohol consumption is embedded in their routine to suddenly stop so consuming, and as the nature of all inner-developmental disciplines is one of continuity and constancy of practice, it would seem far wiser in this day and age to suggest that if you are going to use substances it would be more beneficial to simultaneously continue in your fully mindful state here, than not to.

Obviously it would be best to derive all the mind-altering you require on a daily and nightly basis from the chemically unenhanced methods described here or elsewhere, and perhaps with practice this will naturally come to be the case.

But in the meantime, if you're inclined to indulge in or are required for religious or cultural reasons to ingest mind-altering substances, at no time do so to the extent that you even momentarily obliterate your sense of proper inner assemblage.

No matter how drunk or off your face you may get, always remain fundamentally situated in your three inner chambers, witnessing from the upper, feeling from the middle and driving the experience from the lower. Always remember that the choice between warrior and headless chicken mode is in your hands. Always ensure maximum mainframe expansion and, above all, keep breathing.

Make full use of all previously described inner commands if tripping out of control on acid or stronger and remember you dictate the outcome of any experience with your initial intention.

Interestingly, you will find that by staying mindful while engaged in potentially self-destructive pursuits, your desire to perpetuate the perusal of such self-destruction will diminish of itself over time.

But let us not overlook one of the main reasons we as a species consume such copious quantities of alcohol and drugs, which is to help us immerse ourselves in the following.

CELEBRATION OF LIFE

Obviously life is the most precious 'thing' in the world. Life, this precious, mysterious substance, which can be called the 'Tao' or 'chi' if you want to be more specific, is what you're here to celebrate.

And you don't need to confine this to festival days in the annual calendar, or even – blasphemy of blasphemies – to the variously designated old-school Sabbath days. It is perfectly permissible and highly recommended to celebrate life each and every day from now on, regardless of that day's so-called official designation. In fact, I strongly suggest you extend your self-disciplinary powers to celebrating life each and every moment of every day (and night – even while you dream) for the rest of your life, however long (or short) that might be, from now on.

Forgetting to do so, no matter how difficult the external conditions at the time, is to lose perspective – to lose that moment, in other words. And moments being all you have, you don't want to go around losing them willy nilly all over town.

Every day is a holiday (the word itself a bastardization of holy day), or is if you deem it so. Certainly with all the foregoing (metaphysical) information spinning in your circuits, every day (and night), from now on, is potentially sanctified. And the events that fill those moments are holiday activities, no matter how routine, humdrum, mundane or materially inclined. Even attending to the most irksome detail is an event happening in a moment of your life – which may be your last, you never know – and so worthy of celebration.

However, in case you are misled into assimilating this on a purely abstract level, as just pleasant, reassuring, 'oh yeah!' faux-spiritual blandishment, thus missing its point entirely, let me remind you that the true expression of celebration is dance.

Now of course the action of taking yourself out to a party and 'shakin ya booty' on the dance floor on a regular basis, is one of the best health and wellbeing inducers known to humankind. My god, people have been dancing since the first time someone spontaneously started banging out beats on a log (way before computers knew how to quantize a kick drum pounding four to the floor).

Not only in the electric womb of the ballroom, but also in the privacy of your own home, with suitably chosen soundtrack, allow yourself a private shimmy whenever you get the chance.

But if, as is usually the case, especially in the working urban environment, breaking out into spontaneous dance and showing off your step is inappropriate, it is equally as effective, if not more so, to continue the dance internally by performing (or allowing to be performed) a series of micro movements, or movements within your skin.

Those Taoist dirty dancers of old recommended that you attempt to stand perfectly still for 3 minutes, without moving (or allowing to move) a single strand of a single muscle (other than those used in connection with cardiovascular and respiratory functions), as if possessed of the stoicism and inertness of a large piece of granite.

They suggested that you would soon find this to be impossible. Because life – or chi if you want to nitpick – has movement as its intrinsic quality. Hence nothing that lives (and that includes you, baby) can enter the fully inert state, not even the greatest yogi, fakir or illusionist.

If you were to try now to lock your mainframe into absolute stasis, you too would soon become conscious of small stirrings and promptings from your hips ('Wiggle me, wiggle me!'). You would feel your shoulder blades wanting to gently rotate in alternating directions. You'd want to lift your arm and flex your wrist. In short you'd want to move.

Now if you were to contain that urge so that rather than find expression externally it would do so internally, within the skin of your physical mainframe, undetectable to the naked onlooking eye, you would, if appropriately internally aspected, find yourself giving issue to a complex array of interweaving inner gyrations and omnidirectional, cavorting undulations that extend to inform all parts of your physical mainframe with the ecstasy (literally non-stasis) of the dance.

Tuning in, you can feel it now, gyrating in the back of your neck, moving in a variety of loops of infinite sizes, shapes and speeds through the entire spectrum of multidimensional internal mainframe planes and directions. It's like a hypersonic dragon of invisible light from on high that knows no inner bounds and is dancing the wild fandango for all it's worth, with near reckless abandon, in a series of startling loops that would make a less internally assembled person get dizzy. While as you go casually about your business, from the outside you appear as still as a rock in a lake. (You funky urban warrior, you.)

You can direct micromovement to any part of your mainframe at will and it will serve to cleanse that part of any energetic impurities (blockages will be cleared in other words). This is particularly helpful in the self-treatment of disease. Micromovement is, essentially life or chi in action and is as such a harnessable force to be used for self-healing. But don't let the thought of healing conjure up images of sobriety or dullness. Healing is what you get when you celebrate life or chi in the dance.

Allowing yourself the pleasure of this internal dance on a regular basis will prepare and prime you from the inside for the next time you find yourself on the dance floor and want to immerse yourself fully without the intrusion of unnecessary self-consciousness or uncomfortable outbreaks of unexpected wallflower syndrome.

YOUR ADDICTION TO MORE

You want more, don't you! More text. More ways to grasp the precious jewel of life. More money. More ways of getting high. More sex. More orgasms. More success. More possessions. More friends. More adventure. More excitement. More security. More enlightenment. More fulfilment. More achievements. More tea (or whatever). And more time.

And that in itself is an addiction: wanting more. It is in fact the addiction of all addictions (meant both ways).

No matter the substance or manifestation of what you (think you) want more of, these are merely symptomatic of the mother addiction of wanting more (full stop).

Yet you have found, Pm sure, that in the case of, say, cream cakes, more leads to nausea. You can apply the cream cake test to anything you (think you) want more of. Ultimately, in sufficient quantity, everything is nauseating, no matter what.

Wanting more (and wanting it now) is endemic. It is fueled by impatience and arises from a misguided belief in the exclusivity of linear reality. Believing yourself to be playing an end-game results in fundamental existential confusion about the nature of abundance.

The linear model implies an inherent scarcity of everything you think you want, giving rise to fear of being without (deprivation anxiety), which gives rise to greed. Greed in turn gives rise to scrabbling about, impatiently trying to get as much of what you think you want as you can before the game ends. At which point you lose it all. Clever game. (Not.)

So what do you do? What do you do, as a post-modern urban warrior in a globally urbanized world, to sublimate this impatient, misguided urge to splurge away your remaining moments in such pointless pursuit and yet still maintain a viable life-support system, capable of supplying all resources required to maintain an ongoing physical existence here?

Nothing.

It's not a matter of doing something extra, something more, but of doing something less.

Specifically, do less of looking at life in terms of the linear end-game model, and allow your mind its due luxury of remembering that you exist in a multidimensional lateral, as well as linear, field and that there are no straight lines anyway. Everything returns to its starting point eventually.

With your mind thus opened, it is easier to see how all your needs are in fact met from moment to moment. And if you stop judging situations in which you find yourself as being either good or bad, if you stop holding preferences in other words, and simply surrender to your particular Tao as it is at this moment, welcoming equally whatever comes, with innate equanimity and largesse, everything that happens is groovy (dig?).

Hold no expectations whatsoever other than for life to continue to be magnificent and all-encompassing, and you will not suffer disappointment. Hold your intention as to the essential outcome you want, but entertain no expectation as to the precise form that outcome will finally take.

Simply remain open and equanimous to whatever is going to present itself next.

To help discipline yourself to do this, simply repeat habitually, as if talking to the big friendly Tao itself (or other personified deitific version of your choice), 'What next? (lordy, lordy, what next?!)'

RE-ENTRY

It is common for a hypnotherapist, or someone conducting a trance, to return his or her subject to so-called normal waking reality, by employing a system of counting a progression of numerals in sequential order, either upwards or downwards, as in counting down a rocket launch or counting up from one to ten.

Prior to commencing such countdown or 'count up', he or she would suggest to his (or her) subject that on the pronouncement of a particular numeral towards the end of the series, say either eight or two, you as the subject would feel fully wide awake and back here in the present with me (or he or she).

Not only would you be fully wide awake and here in the present moment with me (or he or she), you'd be feeling more positive, more confident, more self-assured, more spiritually aware, more financially adroit, more successful, more sexy, more desirable, more beautiful, more relaxed, more satisfied, more motivated, more healthy, possessed of more stamina and generally feeling more splendid and glorious than you'd ever thought possible.

But having just explained how more can often turn out to be less and vice versa, and furthermore not being, in this instance, a hypnotherapist conducting you out of a trance, but an author coming (albeit reluctantly) to the end of his (and not 'or her') treatise, I am not confined by such sequential systems.

No ma'am (or man).

I will, however, suggest that on my mention of the number 'nine', your unconscious mind will instantaneously process all the foregoing information (if it feels like) to be made use of as it sees fit, and that you will (probably) feel like reading to the very last page, imbibing such items of interest as grab your fancy as you pass along the text that contains them, and upon reaching the very last word, will close the book, knowing that you can return whenever you like to make more sense of it, and feel pretty damn good about things thereafter (for evermore).

But why, you'd be excused for wanting to know, would I use that particular numeral, not only as the preceding trigger for your smooth re-entry, but as you'll have noticed, in more than a few other instances in connection with the various numbers of repetition of certain exercises, etcetera?

Well, I'll tell you.

THE MYSTERIOUS PROPERTIES OF 'NINE' AND ITS RELATIONSHIP TO THE 'EIGHT', 'SEVEN' AND 'SIX' (IN ITS IMMEDIATE PRECESSION)

All great philosophical schools employ various systems of numerology – the use of numerals as metaphysical symbols, each imbued with its own particular significance – and Taoism is no exception. Indeed, it was from this belief in the sacred power of numbers that the study of mathematics, the purest of all metaphysical studies, developed and upon which all our technological knowledge is based.

According to those particular ancient Orientals, of all the numbers in existence, 'nine' is the most powerful and rich in creative force, yang in other words. 'Six', on the other hand, was considered to be the most diminishing, or yin. And it is indeed a notable coincidence that if you were to position 'six' and 'nine' so as to form a circle with an 'S' running through it, you would in fact be describing exactly the infamous yin-yang symbol itself.

For this reason, 'six' would be used as the number of repetitions of a certain movement to reduce energy in a certain part of the body. Say, for example, you wished to reduce the sudden onset of an unwelcome flow of diarrhoea, you would massage your belly (anticlockwise to back the flow up) six times, the significance of 'six' being its assumed talismanic ability to reduce energy. But say, for example, you wanted instead to clear an unwelcome bout of constipation, you would in fact massage your belly (in a clockwise direction in line with the proposed motion of the large intestine), nine times, the significance being that the power of 'nine' (or yang) would facilitate the creation of an energetic charge that would stimulate the desired internal movement.

And it's interesting to note that when you 'do your nine times table', the individual digits that comprise the resulting multiples throughout the entire sequence form, when added, equal nine. No other number has this property.

Furthermore, it is interesting to note that the individual digits comprising the various multiples throughout the sequential progression follow an exact pattern, which reverses itself at the precise moment you multiply nine by six (mix the yin and the yang in other words), as follows: 1x9=09 (0+9=9); 2x9=18 (1+8=9); 3x9=27(2+7=9); 4x9=36 (3+6=9); 5x9=45 (4+5=9).

Watch the 'six' and how its introduction to the mix causes the digits comprising the various following multiples to reverse their own order, in sequence: 6x9=54 (5+4=9); 7x9=63 (6+3=9); 8x9=72 (7+2=9); 9x9=81 (8+2=9); 10x9=90 (9+0=9). (At'11', the properties of 'nine' enter into an exponential phase fit only for further examination by those possessed of such mathematical skills or urges and beyond the current relevance of this particular item.)

This indicates to some extent why Hendrix, among others, was right to make a fuss about it.

'Six' and 'nine' also often appear (in the Taoist tradition for counting repetitions of exercise movements for instance) in multiples of four, to imbue the 'six' or 'nine' with the turning power of the four seasons.

Meanwhile a certain romantic attachment has always existed, Taoistically speaking, to 'eight' and 'seven', both for their bridge-forming function linking yin with yang (six with nine) and because they are powerful numerals in their own rights, though rarely used for counting repetition purposes.

'Eight', being intrinsically infinite in shape, is thought therefore to symbolize infinity and its scaled down local version, longevity. Thus its properties are considered to contain the power of prosperity, on the basis that situations require time before they yield a profit and must endure if that profit is to be sustained. This is why successful Oriental businessmen like to start new business operations on the eighth of the month and why rich little old Chinese ladies, or indeed big young ones, like to live at an address, have a phone number or drive a car and preferably all three, whose number includes an 'eight' somewhere – preferably standing alone or next to another one or two of its own – it indicates they will thereby prosper.

'Seven', on the other hand, was thought by the Taoists to symbolize completion. This is also the case in Hindu and Buddhist schools, relating as it does to the seven 'chakras' (spinning wheels of psychic energy situated along the equivalent of your penetrating channel, as if you didn't know), as well as to Western schools, based on the idea of the seven days of the week it metaphorically took the creative force to complete its manifestation process (of the universe as we know and love it).

Repetitions of 'seven' tend to be used by more Buddhistically influenced schools, but you can always see a 'seven' appearing somewhere in the action as indicating that a phase has reached or is about to reach completion.

Which, so saying, it nearly has. Not just in terms of us completing a phase of evolution as a species, but also more importantly, as far as you (and of course, I) are concerned at this very moment, in terms of finishing this book.

BEFORE COMPLETION

It is usual to feel anxiety to some degree before any parting, for which all that is necessary is to keep breathing until the anxiety passes, which it surely will (just like everything else in the universe), no matter how momentous the parting, nor from whom you are making such parting.

Every so-called end, as previously discussed, at the risk of stating the obvious, is followed instantaneously by a new beginning. And the only thing that can limit the possibilities of what that brings (you), is this ...

YOUR OWN IMAGINATION

You will have no doubt noticed that you have been required often throughout the preceding text to use your imagination.

Imagination has had mixed press over the years. Some laud it as the very creative force of existence itself, responsible for all the great advances ever made by humankind, which when harnessed in you, the individual, can give you all the metaphysical information you need to make all your dreams come true. In fact, they would say that your ability to materialize your heart's true desire (in the appropriate form for you) is only limited by the extent to which you are willing to use it (imagination).

Others, meanwhile, view imagination with suspicion, believing it to be a resource better relegated to the ranks of childhood memory and fairies at the bottom of the garden, if you want to get on with the serious business of getting ahead. Trouble is, a head's about all you'll have, as your feeling body beneath it will have gone into permanent hibernation out of sheer boredom long before.

We need imagination to stay alive, not in the world of fairies (or at least certainly not there exclusively), but here amongst the metaphorical nuts and bolts of every day, every-night, postmodern, globally urbanized life. (After all there's only so much TV you can watch without becoming a potato(head).

In fact, those intrepid Taoists of old (and indeed this intrepid one of the new) claimed that imagination was the force by which we could most identify with the Tao and was therefore the 'holiest' force of all. And certainly not something to be ashamed of possessing or using.

This philosophy has happily mushroomed in popularity over the recent years – witness the use of imagination in television advertising, for example – and will soon, hopefully, be in the ascendant. Because to survive the conundrum we've collectively unleashed on our own selves by continuing in the way we have on the planet, we will need an unimaginably huge amount of it (imagination) if we are in some way to prevail.

It's a 'use it or lose it' scenario. Use your imagination and you can, in the methods described in this book or others elsewhere, manifest unlimited possibilities in four-dimensional reality. Lose your imagination and you ... well, you may as well be a slug. (That's how much we love it.)

Meantime with all this talk around of phase-completion and the imminent end of the world as we know it (and love it, though you wouldn't know it to look at us), I need to mention a word or two hundred about prophecy (and you).

PROPHECY AND YOU

In 2030, an asteroid the size of Manhattan and Long Island, combined of whatever inconceivably vast tonnage, will come screaming through the afternoon sky and slam into Earth with such force, it'll probably cause a reversal in the magnetic poles and result in curtains for everyone.

Everyone, that is, who has managed, by serendipity or design, to survive the preceding floods, which will wipe out every low (and medium) lying bit of landmass including all major population centers, leaving La Paz and Denver as just about the only places left where you can get a decent hamburger. Or the preceding devastation by fire of vast tracts of previously inhabited land and population centers caused by unpredictable climatic changes and global war erupting out of the Middle East and engulfing the planet in flames, radiation and deathly toxins. Or the preceding breakdown of global infrastructure and of law and order and ensuing mass famine and drought. Or the simultaneous uncontrolled surges of deadly plague epidemics. Or even endless nights sitting in front of the television waiting for something to happen.

And that'll be that. The end. Goodnight. Sayonara.

It's alright, relax, I'm only kidding.

But the forces of destiny might not be.

Which is why it would be foolish to waste a moment longer not enjoying yourself profoundly and appreciating to the full the utter magnificence of your life on Earth at this precise moment, no matter how difficult or existentially irksome the present conditions.

Instead, use your imagination to lend power to the creative vision of us collectively transcending our present, very real (and if you don't believe me, just you wait and see) crisis and encouraging our species' healthy evolution for the sake of future generations.

Specifically, I would like to suggest we change the prophecy, for nothing is so amenable to change as prophecy, by creating the following, or something better, first in the ether by visualizing it, and subsequently to be made manifest in bang-your-foot-material-reality, within the fullness of time.

There is no greater service you can perform on the planet than lending your energy or that personally charged flow of energy within your internal meta-network of energy super-conduits to healing and thus preserving the life of another.

Now, obviously if you want to develop this skill specifically, it's wise to train somehow in the mechanics of the art. Nevertheless, it is the energy initially transmitted on the etheric plane through conscious intention that creates the template upon which the subject's physical or emotional healing subsequently occurs in real time.

As explained when describing the mechanics and dynamics of the etheric web, this is no less so when applied not just to an individual subject, but to the totality of life on the planet at this time.

So, with mainframe appropriately adjusted and all other preliminaries attended to, visualize before you, suspended majestically in space, the planet Earth, complete with white swirly cloud patterns, blue oceans, green (and beige) landmasses and all manner of living things.

As you gaze upon this (majestic vision) from the sanctity of your upper chamber, let your middle chamber be bursting with love for all you see and let your lower chamber be filled with the drive to co-manifest the conditions in which peace, health, harmony, abundance and enlightenment can flourish (tor everyone who wants it).

How emanate from your core out, a stream of intensified etheric light, rose-gold colored if so inclined, channeled through the center of your chest, as if there were an aperture there. See this stream of light span out in all directions in front of you to envelop (your vision of) the planet. In this (new) envelope, see every living creature, every person, every animal, every fish, every bird, every tree, every plant, every insect, every reptile, every amoeba and every microbe suffused with the healing properties contained in the stream of light (emanating from your core).

See every living creature partake of these healing properties, each according to its needs, subsequently to manifest the appropriate conditions for their healthy growth and that of everyone else.

And that includes you (buddy). So simultaneously be aware that you yourself are currently in situ on that precise planet of your visualization and, as such, are entitled this very moment to the full benefits of your own stream of healing energy.

See yourself living on that planet in health, peace and plenty, in mutual harmony and intelligent co-operation, here and now with all other living beings.

For as you see it, so it shall be, as sure as asteroids is asteroids. And we need that vision to manifest urgently. So thank you.

Not that that would necessarily be good. Or bad.

NOT NECESSARILY GOOD, NOT NECESSARILY BAD

If fox-hunting in the UK is banned, that's bad – if you're a dedicated fox hunter, no matter how much others may judge you to be a wanker for it. If you're a fox, who thrives on not being hunted, on the other hand, it's good. Very good.

If the US economy falls into rapid decline, that's bad. (Everyone 'knows' that.) If, that is, you're most of the world's population. If, however, you are in that small cushioned minority, known collectively as bankruptcy specialists, it's good. Damn good, and you'll clean up in no time.

If the prima ballerina twists her ankle and can't do the star turn tonight, that's bad – if you're her or the ballet director. If you happen to be her understudy, however, it's your lucky break (good, in other words).

And if you are that understudy and you shine tonight and get spotted by a rival ballet director, poached and given prima ballerina post, that's good.

But if the sudden increase of pressure on your nervous system is too much for you to handle and you resort to taking pain-killers or other substances to bolster your nerve, that's bad.

But if, during your obligatory stay in rehab, you were to meet someone and the two new reformed yous were to run off hand in hand into the sunset to live happily ever after, that would be good. But if you were the director of the ballet that employed you, that would be bad.

If you were the ballerina's lawyer, however, that would be good, or at least business as usual.

And I must stop that now before it runs away with me to the land of shadows and gets stuck in the realms of relativity for evermore.

Good and bad are not constants. Good and bad are relative terms. Once, however, you delude yourself into believing the opposite to be true, which goodness knows we all do too easily, once you start believing that what you believe is bad is bad no matter what perspective you're looking from, or that what you think is good is so no matter what, then you are making it very difficult for enlightenment to dawn (for you).

A post-modern urban warrior living in a globally urbanized world must greet everything with equanimity if he or she is to maintain himself or herself at optimum inner and outer performance levels when out on the street and otherwise.

There are too many things happening per second to do differently. If you were to judge each one as either fixedly, permanently good or bad, you would quickly become so encumbered by the weight of the judgements you were carrying around, you wouldn't be able to spot or respond to a proper opportunity if it came and head-butted you in the forehead. (Which would be bad. Unless of course you were that opportunity and were possessed of an irrepressible hunger for head-butting unenlightened, prejudiced, bigoted, arrogant know-it-alls in the fore-head. Then it would be good, damn good, or at least would feel damn good at the time).

So yes, of course it's good to develop spiritual, interdimensional, omnipresent, omniscient, omnipotent awareness and with that awareness help heal or at least attempt to heal your world. What finer mission could one undertake? But if you wish to maintain and preserve that privileged, enlightened state in the face of the daily and nightly storm of startling information that constantly assails you, you must be able, without effort or contrivance, to discipline yourself to greet all phenomena, people, events and situations with equanimity.

You train yourself to inwardly respond to all events, no matter how relatively good or bad they first appear, with 'not necessarily good, not necessarily bad'.

This doesn't make you a killjoy. Far from it. It just means you have the wisdom to suspend judgement long enough for that immutable law of yin and yang to take effect so you can see what you're actually dealing with before pronouncing hysterically, 'Good!' (or, 'Bad!').

What is good, and this is not relative (unless you're a murdering, raping, psychotic, twisted person in the position and with the inclination to give effect to those tendencies, but then who am I to judge?), is remembering to breathe, with optimum fluidity, evenness and depth, to ensure maximum vertical and horizontal mainframe expansion and muscular relaxation and sunkenness, and optimum inner assemblage in your three inner chambers, thus facilitating unobstructed passage of energy (the subtle breath) throughout your entire internal meta-network of energy super-conduits for full spirit body identification, at all times no matter what presents itself (for the rest of your life).

What is bad, is not to. Unless of course you want to remain miserable during one of the most exciting phases of human history ever (in the whole wide world.)

To help you remember, place a free palm, preferably your dominant one, across your solar plexus (your upper abdomen) and let the growing warmth penetrate and permeate the entire region, reminding you to keep your diaphragm (large horizontal muscle the alternating contraction and relaxation of which produce the bellow-like action of your lungs), working smoothly. This is especially useful when facing up to any new onslaught of information (the receipt and assimilation of which will give cause for internal and external readjustments to be made, say while talking on an important business or personal phone call, or at a crucial business meeting or love-affair ending (or beginning), or being pulled over by the police in your car, for example).

There's nothing particularly odd-looking about this particular form of palm placement and you'll find you can get away with it on all kinds of occasions, including (boring, let's finally admit it) cocktail parties, especially those where the background music is (oafishly) turned up too loud and you have to engage in mutual eardrum shattering in order to conduct what will probably amount to a meaningless exchange. It will remind you to remember to pay attention to your proper inner assemblage and thus retain your composure as the blood trickles down over your collar.

If, however, you find the conversation taking a turn for the worst and some instant mental action is needed to limit the scale of resulting damage (to whichever aspect of your life that particular conversation is appertaining to), you might like to rest a forefinger on the notch formed at the top of your breastbone and the base of your throat, and gently exert a down-ward pressure, as if trying to make your breastbone slide down your front a centimeter or two. This will have the effect of instantly clearing your head and afford you a more 'grounded' clarity about the situation under discussion. It will also encourage a more considered approach to putting across your viewpoint, as this point controls your throat energy, which in turn controls your ability to communicate.

It will also immediately put you in mind of your correct internal situation (or lack of it) and enable you to make adjustments accordingly.

For this, after all, is the aim of this book: to leave you feeling fully inwardly assembled in the correct manner to be able to meet everyone and everything that comes your way, from now on, with enough composure not to become inwardly or outwardly disheveled and thus incapable of delivering your best performance in the moment (from moment to moment forevermore).

This in turn will lend you a whole new angle on the idea of karma altogether.

Talking of which ...

KARMA! WHAT KARMA!

A young disciple, in love with a beautiful woman who was married to somebody else, but who had intimated her desire for an illicit liaison, went inwardly inflamed with desire and all in an existential tiz, to his master and asked, 'Master, if I were to have an affair with a married woman at this relatively committed stage of my spiritual development, would it be bad karma!'

The master fell into silent contemplation. After some minutes like this, he looked up and in reply, asked, 'How do you know it wouldn't be bad karma not to?' (That put me in a spin I can tell you.)

What the master was saying was, 'Who do you think you are, with your limited local perspective no greater than that of an ant, to presume to understand or even question the workings of something so great and interdimensionally universal in scope as karma?'

Karma, a much misused Hindi word, (often mistaken for 'calmness' or the aroma of incense lingering in someone's hair but meaning the visible workings of the immutable law of cause and effect, when seen in perspective of the infinite rounds of birth and death that both the Hindus and Buddhists believe we undergo before achieving self-realization), does not follow the primitive 'ner, ner, ner, ner-ner' pattern of crime and punishment many in the West believe it to.

The pattern it follows is a matter big enough for only gods to understand, and only then in limited fashion and to the extent that they, like you, have learned to suspend judgement as to what's specifically, inherently bad and what's specifically, inherently good.

Another time, when questioned on the workings of karma, the master retorted, 'Karma? What karma?'

Meaning karma, at the deepest level of the concept, is in reality no more than that: a concept, a belief in a certain implicit order. And as any enlightened soul will tell you, to take your beliefs too seriously, in the knowledge that you shape your internal and hence external conditions by them, is potentially to limit your reality to almost sinful proportions.

Moreover, with no attachment to outcome being either good or bad, being without preferences, in other words, karma ceases to have any significance. This does not mean you don't pay the price of your actions, it simply means you don't take the process personally. (At least I think that's what he meant, but he's dead now, so we'll never know for sure.)

One thing we do know for sure, though, is when you're willing to suspend judgement and welcome whatever's coming next with a childlike 'What's next?', while simultaneously adjusting all internal factors to facilitate optimum interdimensional awareness at all times, you're pretty much guaranteed to have yourself the perfect trip every time. In consideration of which ...

THE PERFECT TRIP

To have the perfect trip, you first have to be willing to believe that whatever happens on the trip is perfect. Then the trip feels so flattered it starts showing off to you and you find you're having a perfect trip. If you spend the whole time getting pissed off that everything isn't perfect, perfection gets offended and withdraws.

And now, if you're feeling settled and secure in the knowledge that everything you've just read (or at least those portions that your discriminating unconscious has chosen not to reject), is now actively spinning its own merry way in a series of improbably elegant micro movements around your internal meta-network of eight energy super-conduits and three internal chambers, and as a result, you'll never be the same again (you wouldn't have been anyway – things change of themselves). I'd just like to say that I hope that, in some small way, I've managed to impart the keys to toning those changes more to your liking.

AND NOW, FINALLY

All that remains to be said, is thank you. Thank you for your time and attention, which we know is important to you. That's why we appreciate your choosing Barefoot Doctor, and hope you'll fly with us again in the future.

It was my intention all along that reading this book would fill you with optimism there and then (here and now) – and pure on-the-spot joy – for what could be better?

If, however, you were to optimize the informational resource offered herewith, you would, as well as being able to legitimately consider yourself to be an urban warrior, also potentially reach that stage of inner development commensurate with the title 'Golden Immortal', possibly just in time for me to write, 'A Modern Manual for Golden Immortals' (working title).

Either way, may it serve you well.

May the Tao take all your troubles away. (May the Tao take everyone's troubles away.) May the Tao always put fine food on your table, etcetera, etcetera (my English teacher, by the way, told me never to use 'etcetera' like that, so fuck you, Mrs Reeves!).

And just one final word of advice: if anyone ever asks you to voluntarily have an electronic chip of any description inserted anywhere within your physical mainframe, no matter how much the prevailing social trends may dictate otherwise at the time, do not, under any circumstances, agree to have it so inserted. Once you do, and believe me it's coming to that, 'they'll' be able to track every move you make, whether your mobile is switched off or not.

And that could seriously alter the internal (and external) dynamic of your moment-to-moment experience of life, in ways you might find decidedly irksome. Always remain chip-free wherever and whenever possible.

Once again, it's been a pleasure talking to you. Thank you for your time. Love, peace, freedom and splendor, Barefoot Doctor.

Also by Barefoot Doctor

'The Tao of Sexual Massage' with Jurgen Kolb, Gaia Books (1992)

'Barefoot Doctor's Handbook for the Urban Warrior' (1998) *also published as 'Barefoot Doctor's Guide to the Tao: A Spiritual Handbook for the Urban Warrior' (1999)*

'Barefoot Doctor's Handbook for Heroes' (1999)

'Barefoot Doctor's Handbook for Modern Lovers' (2000)

'Liberation' (2002) republished as 'Liberation From Your Madness' (2017)

'Instant Enlightenment' (2004)

'Manifesto' (2005) republished as 'Tao of Manifestation' (2017)

'Dear Barefoot: The Wisdom of the Barefoot Doctor' (2005)

'Invincibility Training' (2006)

'Pure' (2008)

'The Man Who Drove With His Eyes Closed' (2009) *also published as 'Supercharged Taoist: An Amazing True Story to Inspire You on Your Own Adventure'' (2010)*

'Jewels of Enlightenment' Nightingale Conant (2009) (audio)

'The Message, vision for a new golden era' (2012)

'Awakening the Laughing Buddha within' (2013) with Joe Hoare

To purchase any of the above, and more, go to

waywardpublications.com

For more on Barefoot Doctor – wisdom drops, events etc. visit

barefootdoctorglobal.com

CPSIA information can be obtained
at www.ICGtesting.com
Printed in the USA
LVHW040018100919
630542LV00006B/342/P

9 781912 062348